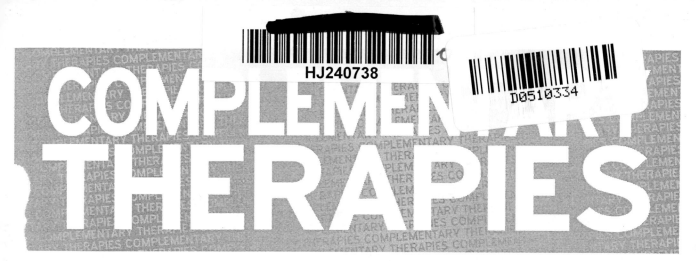

COMPLEMENTARY THERAPIES

The Essential Guide

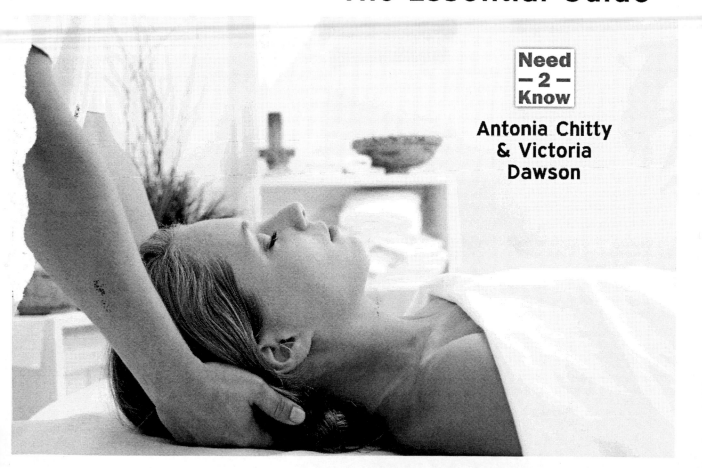

Need
— 2 —
Know

**Antonia Chitty
& Victoria
Dawson**

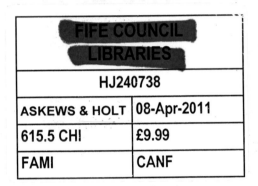
First published in Great Britain in 2011 by
Need2Know
Remus House
Coltsfoot Drive
Peterborough
PE2 9JX
Telephone 01733 898103
Fax 01733 313524
www.need2knowbooks.co.uk

Need2Know is an imprint of Bonacia Ltd.
www.forwardpoetry.co.uk

Contents

Introduction

Do you want to find out more about complementary therapies? Are you looking for an alternative way to relax? Or do you have an illness that you are looking to manage more effectively?

If you are trying to piece together information about complementary therapies, this book is for you. This practical guide is full of information about a range of complementary therapies and packed with case studies from people that have used them.

Sometimes it can be confusing knowing where to start with the different therapies on offer. This book will help you to find out more about the most common complementary therapies currently in use and how they may benefit you or your family.

More and more people in the UK are turning to complementary therapies in order to relieve stress, relax or help some form of illness. The book looks at the most commonly used complementary therapies in detail, covering all aspects, from their history to what you might expect at a consultation. Each chapter covers a different therapy and includes advice from experts about issues such as how to find a suitably qualified practitioner and who the therapy may be useful for.

What is complementary therapy?

Complementary therapy, or alternative therapy as it is sometimes called, is a term used to describe a range of treatments that treat the individual in a holistic way. By this we mean that the whole person is treated, not just the symptom that is troubling them. The belief is that a person is well if their body, mind and environment are all balanced. If, for example, you suffer from migraines, a complementary therapist would look at treating your whole body, your lifestyle, your diet and any mental stress that you are under to ensure that the whole body is working as efficiently as possible. Complementary therapists may also suggest you change your lifestyle.

Medical matters

Complementary therapy is not a substitute for medical advice. If you are ill it is important that you consult your GP. Many doctors now recognise the benefits of complementary therapy; you should discuss your intention to see a complementary therapist with your medical practitioner. You should always continue to take any prescribed medication as instructed by your GP. If you are pregnant or breastfeeding you should always inform the therapist.

Finding a therapist

It is important that you find a suitably qualified therapist. In each chapter we will give you tips to help you to find a professional and reputable therapist. You should check that the therapist is insured and ask to see proof of their qualifications. You may also wish to ask the therapist about their experience and whether they have treated people with a similar condition to yours before.

You should choose a therapist that you feel comfortable with. It is important that you have confidence in their abilities. Word of mouth is often a good way of finding a therapist.

If you are taking a child to a therapist you should establish what experience they have working with children. You should check that you are able to stay with your child throughout the treatment. If your child is older and wishes to receive the treatment alone, then you should ask whether the therapist is CRB (Criminal Records Bureau) checked.

When receiving a treatment you should feel comfortable in the surroundings. You should expect the room to be clean, uncluttered and have a relaxing ambience.

Cost

While some complementary therapies are beginning to become available on the NHS, it is usual to expect to pay for treatments privately. You should find out about the cost of the treatment prior to booking an appointment. It is also advisable to ask the therapist how many sessions you are likely to need so that you have some idea of the cost prior to committing to the therapy. You may also wish to ask about whether there is a discount for block booking a number of treatments. If you have private medical insurance it is worth checking your policy to see if it covers any complementary therapies.

Regulations and complementary therapies

The Complementary and Natural Healthcare Council (CNHC) is the only UK regulatory body for complementary healthcare. Their contact details can be found in the useful contact section at the end of this book. CNHC is endorsed and supported by the Department of Health who encourage practitioners to register. It was established in 2008 and opened its register to various complementary healthcare disciplines during 2009. Its purpose is to protect the public by means of a voluntary register for complementary and natural healthcare practitioners.

CNHC currently registers practitioners who meet its standards in aromatherapy, Alexander Technique, Bowen therapy, massage therapy, nutritional therapy, reflexology, shiatsu, sports and remedial and yoga therapy. At the time of publication the CNHC were opening the register to more disciplines, including cranial sacral therapy, naturopathy, reiki, hypnotherapy, Microsystems Acupuncture and healing. For the latest information please visit the CNHC website at www.cnhc.org.uk.

The CNHC has a number of functions including:

- To establish and maintain a voluntary register of complementary healthcare practitioners in the UK who meet its standards of competence and practice.

- To make the register of practitioners available to the general public.

- To educate the public about the CNHC quality mark as a quality standard.

- To operate a robust process for handling complaints about registered practitioners.

- To work with professional bodies in the complementary healthcare field to further develop and improve standards of professional practice.

Unregulated complementary therapy professions are encouraged by the government to develop their own unified systems of voluntary self-regulation. Details of any self-regulatory organisations are included in each chapter.

Summary

It is estimated that around 30% of the population in the UK use complementary therapy and this figure continues to rise. Complementary therapies can provide you with some quality time away from the stress of everyday life. They may also help you to manage an illness more effectively. Complementary therapies can be used by the young and old alike and many women turn to complementary therapy during pregnancy. Each chapter explores who may benefit from the therapy and any contraindications that you may need to be aware of before booking a treatment.

If you are unsure where to start with the different therapies on offer, read on to find out more about the most common complementary therapies currently in use and how they may benefit you or your family.

Disclaimer

This book is for general advice on complementary therapies and isn't intended to replace medical advice. It can be used alongside medical advice but you should discuss your intention to see a complementary therapist with your health practitioner before undertaking treatment.

Chapter One

Acupuncture

Acupuncture involves the insertion of very fine needles under the skin at specific points on the body to free the flow of energy or 'qi' (pronounced 'chee'). Acupuncturists treat each person individually as each case is unique. They believe that illness and pain only occur when the body's vital energy (qi) cannot flow freely. This blockage can occur for a number of reasons, including stress, diet, injury or emotional difficulties.

Acupuncture is considered to be very safe. Two surveys were conducted in 2001 and published in the *British Medical Journal*. They concluded that the risk of severe adverse reaction to acupuncture is less than 1 in 10,000. Acupuncture has very few side effects when carried out by a qualified practitioner and all members of the British Acupuncture Council (BAcC) observe a code of safe practice which lays down stringent standards of hygiene and requires the use of sterile disposable needles.

To understand how acupuncture works, it is important to be aware of its principles. The Chinese believe that 'qi' flows through every living being and is responsible for life. This energy flows through the body through what are referred to as 'meridians'. These meridians influence different organs, so for example there is a meridian that influences the heart and another that influences the lungs and so on. Some of the meridians are negative and some are positive in orientation, these are referred to as the 'yin' and 'yang'. The yin meridians include hollow organs, such as the stomach, the intestines and the bladder. The yang incorporate solid organs, like the heart, lung, liver and kidneys.

The belief is that if a person is healthy the yin and yang are in equilibrium and energy will flow through them equally. However, in a person that is ill, less energy will flow through the meridians and the yin and yang will become unbalanced. Acupuncture works by clearing the obstruction and allowing the energy flow to be restored which helps the person to become healthy again.

Needles are inserted at different depths depending on the area being worked on, a skilled practitioner, however, should be able to insert the needles without you feeling any pain. You may feel a dull sensation where the needles are inserted. After the session you may be able to see slight pinprick-sized marks where the needles have been, but usually there is no lasting redness or marking of the skin. Sometimes there may be slight bruising at the site of insertion.

Acupressure, like acupuncture, stimulates pressure points and meridians. The difference is that acupressure does not use needles. The therapist uses their fingers and other parts of their body to skilfully apply pressure to the required areas. Acupressure can be taught and used at home, there are a number of books and instructional DVDs available on the market if it is something that you wish to learn more about.

History

Acupuncture is steeped in history; it emerged from the Far East around 2,500 years ago. The first needles used were reportedly made from stone. Later gold, silver and bronze were used, today the needles are made from steel. Acupuncture was documented in *The Yellow Emperor's Classic of Internal Medicine*, which is dated at around 300 BC.

During the 1970s, traditional Chinese medicine was given new opportunities to develop. Acupuncture continues to be used extensively in China where it is practised in hospitals alongside conventional medicine.

Physicians and missionaries introduced acupuncture into Europe in the 17th century. A journalist for the *New York Times* called James Reston was responsible for spreading the word about the therapy in the West. He had been given acupuncture when he had an emergency appendectomy while in China in 1972. Acupuncture is now gaining popularity across the globe and is practised throughout the world.

A typical treatment

Your first treatment will take longer than subsequent treatments as the practitioner will want to take a full history of your case. You can expect to be asked about your diet, sleep patterns, emotional state and medical history. The practitioner may wish to examine your tongue, take your pulse and examine you for signs of muscle tension. It is important that you tell the therapist about any medications that you are currently taking.

From this information the therapist will be able to devise a treatment plan. Sometimes they may recommend a change in diet or lifestyle to complement the acupuncture.

After you have told the practitioner about your health and lifestyle, they will insert fine needles at various points of your body to stimulate them. The points where the needles are inserted are not always close to the site of the difficulty. For example, if you are experiencing migraines you may have needles inserted in your feet and hands to help to clear the meridians. The number of needles inserted varies depending on your individual needs. The needles are left in place for a short period of time before being removed, you may enjoy some quiet time listening to relaxing music with the lights dimmed at this point. You should not experience any pain when the needles are either positioned or removed.

You should wear loose clothing for your treatment so that it can easily be moved in order to insert needles.

What is it used for?

Acupuncture can be used for a variety of purposes including:

- Pain relief.
- Headaches.
- Skin problems.
- Bowel difficulties, such as Irritable Bowel Syndrome (IBS).
- Menstrual and fertility problems.
- Stress relief.

Contraindications

There are certain circumstances when acupuncture should not be used. These include:

- Medical emergencies.
- If you have a blood or clotting disorder.
- At the site of tumours.

Use with children

Acupuncture can be used successfully with babies and children. Some therapists specialise in paediatric care which means that they work specifically with children. May Stevens practises acupuncture from her clinic in Sheffield. She tells us, 'In the West, most people are unaware that children can respond extremely well to acupuncture. It has been used for thousands of years in China to treat a wide range of conditions. When treating children, the qualified practitioner will be aware that the points used should be kept to a minimum, around four needles per treatment, that the needles should be left in for a much shorter time than in adults and needling technique should be very gentle. For children averse to needling, techniques such as acupressure and massage can be used instead. If you are considering acupuncture treatment for your child, looking for a practitioner who has a special interest in treating children would be a good thing to do.'

Use with pregnant women

Acupuncture can be safely used by pregnant women throughout all three trimesters. May Stevens says, 'From a properly trained practitioner, acupuncture is a perfectly safe treatment for pregnant women. Many women choose acupuncture for conditions of pregnancy because regular treatments, such as medication from the GP, are not appropriate for them at this time. Conditions that can be helped by acupuncture include morning sickness, aches and pains (e.g. back pain, sciatica or pelvic pain), constipation and heartburn, and acupuncture can even be used to promote the turning of a breech position baby and to induce an overdue labour. Certain acupuncture points are traditionally avoided during pregnancy but your acupuncturist will be well aware of this fact and will tailor their prescription accordingly.'

Use with older people

Older people can also benefit from acupuncture. It can be used very successfully alongside conventional medicine. Some therapists are willing to visit older people at home in order to provide the treatment. This can be helpful for those that are less mobile. Another benefit is that immediately following the treatment you can enjoy a nap without having to worry about getting home. Ask when making an enquiry whether this is an option.

What the experts say

Acupuncturist May Stevens explains what we are likely to experience if we choose to try acupuncture, 'The needling sensation depends, in part, on which acupuncture point the needle is being inserted into. Common descriptions of the sensations produced are "tingling", "warming", "pressure", "aching" or "dullness" but it should not be painful. These sensations are usually a good sign, showing that the acupuncture point has been reached and is being stimulated by the needle.'

Many people can feel worried about having needles inserted, May offers reassuring words, 'Most people's past experience of needles is having an injection or having a blood sample taken using a hypodermic needle. Acupuncture needles are completely different. They are much finer and don't need to be hollow like hypodermic needles, as there is nothing that will be passing through them. Many practitioners now also use plastic guide-tubes around the needles to enable them to be quickly and painlessly tapped through the skin. Most of my patients say that it was much less painful than they were expecting and that it was certainly nothing to be frightened of.'

Log on to May's website at www.maystevensacupuncture.co.uk.

Case study

It can often be helpful to read other people's experiences of therapies. Here, Lucy tells us about how she turned to acupuncture in order to help with fertility issues.

'After months of trying for a baby, with no success, I decided to give acupuncture a try. I am absolutely terrified of needles and often faint if I have to have an injection. The thought of acupuncture was frightening but I was desperate and would try anything. I'd read about fertility issues being helped with acupuncture and a friend who had similar problems got pregnant after giving it a go. I used the same practitioner and felt reassured as she is also a doctor of conventional medicine. I immediately shared my fears about the needles with her and she put me at ease instantly. The therapist took a great deal of time talking to me about my difficulties and also about my lifestyle and emotional wellbeing. Medical investigations had shown that I wasn't ovulating.

'I had to lie down on a bed and the therapist cleansed my skin with surgical spirit where the needles were to be inserted. I had several in my feet, some in my hands and a number in my head with the occasional needle inserted in my stomach. I felt no pain when the needles were tapped into place. In fact what I felt was very strange, I was overcome with this feeling of heaviness and relaxation. I can remember thinking, "I'm never going to be able to get off this bed" as I felt so numb. The needles were left in for about 20 minutes and I actually enjoyed this period of time. The therapist was very efficient at removing them and again this was a pain-free experience. After the treatment I felt incredibly relaxed, in fact I just wanted to curl up and go to sleep. I had around six treatments in total. We were told by the fertility specialists that we couldn't have children and our name was placed on the IVF waiting list. The very same week I found out that I was pregnant! It is very hard to prove that the acupuncture helped with my ovulation but it certainly helped me to feel calmer and more relaxed than I have done for years.'

How to find a practitioner

May advises, 'If you are thinking of having acupuncture, and have not got a recommendation for a particular practitioner from a satisfied friend or acquaintance, then your first port of call should be the British Acupuncture Council. You can be sure that a practitioner registered with the British Acupuncture Council has at least three years' full-time degree-level training and is fully insured to treat you. They will also be obliged to follow strict codes of safety, hygiene and professional conduct. Many practitioners offer free short consultations where they will talk to you about your health concerns. This is a great opportunity to find out whether your chosen practitioner is someone you feel comfortable with and to get their professional opinion of how acupuncture may be able to help.'

The British Acupuncture Council is a self-regulatory body for acupuncture in the UK. It sets out standards of practice in its professional code for therapists to follow. Members are also expected to meet the Council's Code of Safe Practice which ensures that people are treated in a safe manner. You can contact the Council directly to request information about local practitioners, their contact details can be found in the help list.

Quick action checklist

- Consider whether acupuncture is something that you or a member of your family would like to try.
- Ask any friends or colleagues about their experiences with acupuncture.
- Find out more about acupuncture by contacting the British Acupuncture Council.

Summing Up

Acupuncture is a complementary therapy that dates back many years. It can be useful in treating many conditions and has very few contraindications, meaning that it is suitable for most people. If you are interested in looking at research into the effectiveness of acupuncture visit www.acupunctureresearch.org.uk, the research centre has a set of briefing papers that can be reviewed online that review the evidence of the effectiveness of acupuncture treatments for specific conditions.

Chapter Two

Aromatherapy

Aromatherapy is the use of plant oils to promote psychological and physical wellbeing. The oils are collected from plants and are called 'essential oils'. They are extracted from flowers, leaves, roots, peel, bark or resin and there are over 90 essential oils that can be used in aromatherapy. Sometimes an aromatherapist will use oils mixed in combination with carriers, like cold pressed vegetable oils, milk powders or clays and muds. Products that include synthetic ingredients are not used. You may see bottles of fragrance oils on offer in retail outlets, these are not the same as essential oils as they do not provide the same therapeutic benefits.

Aromatherapy can not only be used to promote wellbeing and relaxation, but also to actively treat illness or disease. The products used are usually applied on the outside of the body and are absorbed through your skin. There are a number of ways that this can happen; sometimes the oils are massaged into the skin using a cream, diluted oil or lotion. The oils can also be inhaled.

The gentle massaging of the oils into the skin has a relaxing effect for many people. You can choose to visit an aromatherapist for a full treatment, or you may wish to buy oils to use at home and carry out the treatment yourself. You should always bear in mind that concentrated oils can be very powerful and that you should handle them carefully. Always dilute them according to the instructions and only use externally.

Research into aromatherapy and its effectiveness brings up conflicting results and more research is needed. There is, however, plenty of anecdotal evidence from individuals who use aromatherapy and feel that it works well for them. Some studies have shown that aromatherapy may help to improve the quality of life for people with cancer and reduce feelings of agitation in people with dementia.

History

It is believed that aromatherapy is around 6,000 years old and has been used by many cultures throughout the world. The Ancient Egyptians used oils from plants to treat a range of illnesses. They also used oils in the mummification process, while the Aztecs of South America were also documented as using plants for their aromas. The Romans were well known for taking scented baths and used aromatic oils.

Exotic oils were brought back to Europe during the 16th century and were used to scent handkerchiefs. In France, lavender and rosemary oils were used to fumigate the hospitals. This led to scientists researching the effects of oils on bacteria in the 19th century.

In the 1930s, a French chemist called Dr René-Maurice Gattefossé published his research about the anti-microbial effects of essential oils; he used the term 'aromatherapy'. Another French biochemist, Margaret Maury, developed massage techniques to aid the effective application of essential oils onto the skin. Aromatherapy continues to be popular and more readily available in the 21st century.

A typical treatment

Your first treatment will involve taking a detailed history about your lifestyle, health problems, diet and wellbeing. There should also be the opportunity to ask any questions that you may have. If you think of questions before your appointment make a note of them to remind you what you wanted to ask.

Aromatherapy is a holistic treatment and the therapist will try to find oils that suit you both physically and mentally. If the treatment involves a massage they may mix several oils together to form a blend specifically made for you. The oils will be mixed with what is a called a 'carrier oil'. The carrier oil, bland and neutral in itself, may be made from grapeseed or nuts and helps to carry the essential oils and provide lubrication for the massage. You must ensure that you tell your therapist if you have any allergies, particularly if you are allergic to nuts.

You should ask your aromatherapist how many sessions you are likely to need and what the cost implications are prior to making a booking.

What is it used for?

Aromatherapy can be used for a variety of purposes including:

- Muscular aches.
- Digestive problems.
- Menstrual difficulties.
- Headaches.
- Stress and anxiety.
- Insomnia.

Contraindications

Concentrated oils need to be handled very carefully as they can be extremely potent – neat oils should not be applied directly to the skin without being diluted. Aromatherapy oils should not be used on broken skin or taken internally.

You need to take extra care if you have conditions such as:

- Asthma.
- Eczema or sensitive skin.
- Allergies or hay fever.

Aromatherapy may not be suitable if you have:

- Epilepsy.
- High blood pressure.
- Deep vein thrombosis.

If you are taking medication or have an ongoing health condition you should check with your GP before using aromatherapy. Some essential oils may reduce the effects of conventional medicines, so always seek medical advice.

Use with children

Aromatherapy can be used successfully with children but caution should always be exercised when using essential oils. Always check with a qualified aromatherapist before using oils with your child and make sure that your child is supervised when using oils. There are many oils that should not be used with children. If you are unsure about safety do not use an oil on your child. There are a number of products on the market that use aromatherapy oils and have been especially formulated for use with children. Buying products such as these can help you to ensure their safety.

Use with pregnant women

Aromatherapy can be used during the second and third trimesters of pregnancy but oils should not be directly massaged into the abdomen and some oils should be avoided altogether. Oils should be avoided for the first 12 weeks of pregnancy. A qualified aromatherapist will be able to advise you about which oils are suitable. Some mums-to-be enjoy using aromatherapy at the birth of their child, finding it helps them to relax and stay calm.

As there are specific oils that should be avoided during pregnancy, it is important that you take professional advice before using aromatherapy in pregnancy.

Use with older people

Older people may benefit from using essential oils, although if they are frail they may need the oils to be used in a more dilute form. Elderly people are also more likely to have health problems so it is important that they contact their GP prior to a treatment taking place to ensure that the oils will not contraindicate any medication or condition.

Use at home

You should get advice from a registered aromatherapist before using essential oils at home, but here are some tips to help you:

- Any oils that you use should be diluted.
- Make sure that you read the guidelines and follow the instructions carefully.
- The oils must be stored in a cool, dark place and should be kept out of reach of children.

You can use aromatherapy at home in a number of ways:

- Add a few drops into the bath.
- Inhale the oils by adding a few drops to steaming water.
- Use an oil burner to fragrance a room.
- Add a few drops to unperfumed creams, lotions or shampoos.

Case studies

Roberta tells us, 'I use aromatherapy on a regular basis to help me with stress management. It does help me to relax and seems to take some of life's pressures away so that I can cope a little better. I personally find that aromatherapy works for me and I enjoy every moment of my treatment.'

Joanne uses aromatherapy at home, 'After having a number of sessions with a qualified aromatherapist I decided to start using aromatherapy at home. I only use the blends that she mixes for me as I want to make sure that they are safe. Sometimes I buy a cream from her and use this to massage into my skin. I also enjoy having an aromatherapy bath and believe that it helps me to get a better night's sleep. I think breathing in the oils in the bath while allowing them to soak into my skin really helps them to work more effectively.'

What the experts say

Caroline Preen is the senior consultant aromatherapist from the Aromatherapy Council. She tells us, 'Aromatherapy can treat a wide range of conditions, but legally we cannot make any medicinal claims on essential oils. We can say however that it helps a wide range of acute and chronic symptoms and is great for all stress-related illnesses.'

Sharon Murphy is an aromatherapist and runs Maia Skin Care, a company specialising in natural skincare products. Sharon tells us, 'Aromatherapy offers a natural multi-functional option to skincare products. Many essential oils contain active compounds that are of great benefit to the skin whilst the subtle natural aromas create positive emotions. Maia Skin Care products all contain essential oils to help both balance and revitalise the skin whilst soothing and uplifting the mind. When buying essential oils for use at home make sure you are buying pure therapeutic grade essential oils, not fragrance grade which may contain synthetic chemicals. Although essential oils are natural they are also highly concentrated and potent, so they must always be properly diluted.'

How to find a practitioner

Aromatherapy is now a regulated profession under the CNHC. CNHC is the only voluntary regulatory body for complementary healthcare which has official government backing. Their website details can be found in the help list and includes a section about how to find a practitioner.

Many people find an aromatherapist by word of mouth. If this is the case you should check the training that they have undertaken and that they are fully insured. The Aromatherapy Council website lists recognised qualifications and professional bodies so that you can check your therapist's credentials (see help list).

Quick action checklist

- Look for a qualified practitioner – find a personal recommendation or search the CNHC register.

- Consult a qualified aromatherapist to discuss your needs and suitable oils.
- Investigate products that you can use at home.

Summing Up

Aromatherapy can be used for a range of purposes, and an aromatherapist will work with you to make sure that the oils used are specifically blended to meet your needs. The use of aromatherapy is becoming more and more common; it is now used in the home as well as in clinics, hospitals and even schools. Always be aware that aromatherapy oils can be extremely potent and therefore seek professional advice before using them at home.

Chapter Three

Chiropractic

If you have problems with your joints, ligaments and/or tendons you may wish to consider visiting a chiropractor. The term 'chiropractic' comes from the Greek words, 'cheir' which means 'hand' and 'praktos' meaning 'done'. Chiropractic is: 'A health profession concerned with the diagnosis, treatment and prevention of mechanical disorders of the musculoskeletal system, and the effects of these disorders on the functions of the nervous system on general health. There is an emphasis on manual treatments including spinal adjustment and other joint and soft-tissue manipulation.' World Federation of Chiropractic Dictionary definition, 2001.

Chiropractic involves the use of a range of manipulative techniques which are designed to improve the function of joints and muscle spasms and therefore relieve pain. No drugs or surgery are involved. The chiropractor will refer you to another health care professional if chiropractic treatment is inappropriate for you. Chiropractic is now regulated by the General Chiropractic Council (GCC). Legally, only someone on the GCC register can call themselves a chiropractor. You do not necessarily need to be referred to a chiropractor by your GP. Research supports the use of chiropractic care and some people may be able to access the treatment via the NHS. Discuss this with your GP to see if there is anything available in your area. You can also see a chiropractor on a private basis. Chiropractic is covered by many private health insurers and if you do have a policy make sure that you check it for details.

History

Spinal manipulation dates back thousands of years in Greek and Chinese civilisations. It was Daniel David Palmer, however, who established a chiropractic school, Palmer College in Davenport, Iowa in 1897. At the time the practice was criticised and chiropractors were accused of practising medicine without a licence. Palmer's son, Bartlett Joshua, continued his father's work and is credited with developing chiropractic into the practice that we recognise today. His contribution to research was extensive and he improved methods of spinal adjustment increasing awareness of chiropractic throughout the world.

Chiropractic is the world's third largest primary health care profession and is statutorily regulated in the UK, and has developed rapidly, being practised on every continent.

A typical treatment

Your first appointment is likely to take longer than subsequent appointments. You will usually be asked to complete some paperwork regarding your medical history. Your chiropractor will take time to ask you about your medical history and will answer any questions that you have about your visit. You will be asked about your occupation, medications you're taking and other general questions about your lifestyle. Sometimes it is necessary for X-rays to be taken as an aid to diagnosis and many practices have facilities to do this on site. Like all health care practitioners, the use of X-rays is governed by the Ionising Radiation (Medical Examination) Regulations. This means that you will only be offered X-rays if they are necessary, and your results will be examined by a properly qualified professional.

A physical examination will take place, you should ask the practice what to wear before the appointment, although gowns are provided for your use should you so wish. The chiropractor will examine you in detail and will undertake a range of tests to check your joint and muscle functions.

Treatment may commence at the first session, depending on what is found during the examination. The chiropractor will give you a diagnosis and advise you on the best course of treatment and discuss this with you so that you can understand what will happen. Treatment will only be undertaken once you have given your consent and the benefits and potential side effects of treatment have been explained. Manipulation can be used whereby the chiropractor moves a joint a little further than you would be able to independently. You may hear a 'pop' when you are being manipulated; this is nothing to worry about.

This sound is caused by the small bubbles of gases that are created in the synovial fluid between the joints. Manipulation helps to normalise the functions of the joints or muscles worked on and to alleviate painful symptoms.

The chiropractor may also treat your soft tissues – that means muscles and tendons – and may use massage techniques or stretching. You may also be shown exercises that you can carry out at home to help to take care of your body.

What is it used for?

Chiropractic can be used for the following:

- Back, neck and shoulder pain.
- Poor muscle function.
- Referred pain: this is when badly functioning joints and muscles can cause pain in other areas. For example, a badly functioning shoulder muscle may cause pain in the neck.
- Headaches, migraines and dizziness.
- Sports injuries.
- Leg pain and sciatica.
- Postural difficulties.
- Pain and stiffness related to arthritis and wear and tear, particularly of the hip and knee.

Contraindications

Chiropractic is considered to be very safe. The chiropractor will take a detailed medical history to ensure that there are no contraindications to receiving chiropractic treatment and will explain any risk factors to you.

Use with children

Chiropractic is a safe and effective treatment for babies and children and the techniques used are modified to suit each person's needs. The techniques used are gentle and can be effective at easing symptoms and discomfort. Birth can be a traumatic time for a baby and may result in irritation through spinal and cranial misalignment. More research is needed, but it is thought that these contribute to some of the most common infant health complaints, such as colic, and its associated symptoms of feeding difficulties, sleep problems and ear infections.

Use with pregnant women

With an increase in hormones women find that their ligaments and joints slacken during pregnancy. This can make the joints weaker and can lead to backache and sciatic pain. The growing bump can also add additional strain on the spine. Chiropractic care can help alleviate the musculoskeletal problems associated with pregnancy and is safe for both mother and baby.

Gemma tells us, 'When I was pregnant with my second child I suffered from a condition called "Symphysis Pubis Dysfunction" or SPD for short. It resulted in pelvic pain throughout the pregnancy. When I was around 18 weeks pregnant I was struggling to walk as the pain was so severe. I was on the waiting list to see a physiotherapist when a friend suggested I look into chiropractic as a way of managing the pain. I booked an appointment and had my first consultation. I've got to admit I was a little bit nervous about being manipulated and worried about the impact on the baby. The chiropractor put me at ease and spent a long time talking to me and examining me before she carried out any treatment. I had weekly sessions until I was able to be seen by the physiotherapist and it did give me my quality of life back. I was able to continue working as planned until I was 35 weeks pregnant. The treatment wasn't painful and involved the chiropractor manipulating joints and massaging areas of my back where I had the pain. The initial consultation took about 45 minutes and then after that sessions lasted around 15 minutes each time.'

Use with older people

Older people can also benefit from chiropractic care and may find it particularly helpful to ease aching joints and arthritic pain associated with ageing. The chiropractic techniques used are modified to suit each individual person's needs.

Case study

George has suffered with difficulties with back pain for most of his life. Here he tells us how he has had some relief from visiting a chiropractor on a regular basis.

'I first visited a chiropractor about 20 years ago now. At the time I felt utter despair as conventional medicine just was not helping my condition. I now see a chiropractor on a regular basis to ensure that my back problems do not ever become as chronic as before. Each session lasts about half an hour and consists of the chiropractor manipulating the affected parts. At times I can experience some pain but it is in short bursts and is tolerable. At £25 a session the treatment is relatively expensive but I feel it is worth the cost to be pain-free. I usually visit around once a week until the affected part is stabilised and then I'm seen around every 6 to 8 weeks for monitoring. If others are suffering with pain I would recommend trying to find a chiropractor locally to visit.'

What the experts say

Richard Brown, president of the British Chiropractic Association, says, 'Chiropractic is now very much part of the mainstream approach to effective back care. Although chiropractors are best known for using spinal manipulation, modern practice uses a range of techniques and involves the patient as an active partner in the recovery process with exercises, lifestyle modifications and education.

'It's clear that patients prefer an approach that does not rely upon long-term drug prescription but puts them in control of their wellbeing. For most patients with back pain, staying active and a positive approach to a healthy lifestyle produces best outcomes and chiropractors play an important role in advice as well as treatment. Knowing when to refer is also important and modern chiropractors work closely with GPs and spinal surgeons to help patients achieve the best outcomes.

'The NICE guidelines on lower back pain issued in 2009, endorse the chiropractic approach to managing back pain and NHS providers are now looking seriously at how it can be incorporated into their provision of care for back pain sufferers. This integrated model uses the expertise of a range of specialists so that patients can access the most appropriate treatment.'

How to find a practitioner

The British Chiropractic Association is the largest and longest established association for chiropractors in the United Kingdom. Their website allows you to make a postcode search to find your nearest BCA registered chiropractor, visit www.chiropractic-uk.co.uk. The GCC also has a similar search facility on their website at www.gcc-uk.org. All chiropractors in the UK must be registered with the GCC, they ensure that chiropractors who apply for registration have a suitable qualification and are of sound character and it is illegal to use the title 'chiropractor' unless the practitioner is registered with the GCC. All chiropractors must comply with the GCC's Code of Practice and Standard of Proficiency. The GCC also sets standards of chiropractic education in the UK and deals with complaints, some chiropractors use the honorary title 'Dr' and this is legal as long as they make it clear that they are a registered chiropractor and not a registered medical practitioner.

Some chiropractors have a specialist interest in certain aspects of work, for example treating children or sports injuries. You may find it helpful to ask about any specialist areas that they work in when you phone for an appointment.

Quick action checklist

▪ Check whether a chiropractor you are planning to use is registered with the GCC.

▪ Ask about their specialist interests/areas.

▪ Find out if you have any health insurance that can help to cover the cost of treatment or whether you can receive treatment on the NHS.

Summing Up

Chiropractors can treat a variety of problems and are associated with working with the musculoskeletal system. There are many reasons why problems can occur with the body, including poor posture, illness, lack of exercise and general wear and tear.

A chiropractor will work with you to devise a treatment plan which may involve manipulation and massage, sometimes you will be asked to carry out exercises at home. The treatment is undertaken in partnership with the chiropractor and you should always choose a practitioner with whom you feel comfortable. Make sure that you ask questions if you are unclear about anything to get the most benefit from your treatment.

Chapter Four

Herbal Medicine

In herbal medicine, practitioners treat a wide range of conditions using extracts from plants and herbs. Many herbs are taken orally, some can be in tablet form, tinctures, creams, balms or teas. Herbal medicine uses a holistic approach: this means that the practitioner looks at you as a whole person rather than simply treating a single part of you. A herbal medicine practitioner will assess your general and physical health before starting treatment and can work with you over a period of months or weeks. Herbal medicine is used to treat a range of conditions, including menopause symptoms, irritable bowel syndrome, skin problems and arthritis.

Introduction to herbal medicine

Peter Conway is the president of the College of Practitioners of Phytotherapy and practises in Tunbridge Wells, Kent. He says, 'Herbal medicine is extraordinary – it is the oldest form of medicine and is the origin of conventional medicine. In fact the word "drug" comes from a Teutonic word meaning "a dried plant". After years of neglect this global treasure is now returning to the cutting edge as physiologists and pharmacologists begin to advocate drugs that can affect "multiple targets" in the body – this is what herbs do and which gives them their exceptional scope of therapeutic impact. The herbal approach is known as phytotherapy ("phyto" is Greek for plant), and draws upon the evidence for herbal medicine to integrate traditional and scientific approaches.'

Regulation and safety – practitioners

At time of writing it is proposed that all practitioners supplying herbal medicines to members of the public must be registered with the Health Professions Council by 2012. Registrants are required to meet the HPC's standards of proficiency for safe and effective practice and for continuing professional development.

Herbalists can also choose to become a member of a professional body.

The National Institute of Medical Herbalists (NIMH) is the UK's leading professional body for herbal practitioners. It has a register of individual members and sets educational standards for its members, this requires them to take part in ongoing professional development. Members must comply with codes of conduct, ethics and practice. The NIMH has a complaints process and disciplinary procedures. It requires members to have professional indemnity insurance.

The European Herbal and Traditional Medicine Practitioners Association represents practitioners using Ayurveda, Chinese herbal medicine, traditional Tibetan medicine and Western herbal medicine.

Requirements for insurance and complaints procedures mean that it is safer to choose a practitioner who is a member of such a professional body.

Regulation and safety – remedies

Many herbal remedies can be bought over the counter in health food shops and pharmacies, as well as through catalogues and on the Internet. You can take herbal remedies as:

- Herbal teas.
- Herbal decoctions.
- Herbal syrups.
- Herbal tinctures.
- Infused oils.

- Salves, ointments and creams.

Just because these remedies are 'natural' it does not mean that they are always safe for you to use.

The Medicines and Healthcare Products Regulatory Agency (MHRA) is the government agency which is responsible for ensuring that medicines and medical devices work, and are acceptably safe. It highlights specific concerns about the 'weak regulation of herbal remedies in the UK'. Herbal remedies may be:

- Unlicensed.

- Registered.

- Licensed.

Unlicensed remedies do not have to meet any safety or quality standards and there are no requirements for information on how to use the remedy. Unlicensed remedies are being phased out. From April 2011, all manufactured herbal medicines must have either a traditional herbal registration or a product licence.

Registered remedies must meet specific standards of safety and quality under the Traditional Herbal Medicines Registration Scheme. The product must tell you what it can be used for, based on traditional practice and each product must also be accompanied by information on safe use. You will be able to see the THR certification mark on these products and the letters THR followed by some numerals. The Medicines and Healthcare Products Regulatory Authority explains, 'Where a herbal medicine carries the Certification Mark, this means

 that the MHRA has assessed the product to ensure that it is acceptably safe when used as intended, is manufactured to the quality standards set by the agency, and is accompanied by reliable and accurate product information for the public and patients. The authorised usage and dosage of the medicine is based on evidence of its traditional use. The effectiveness of the product has not been assessed by the MHRA.'

Licensed remedies are subject to the same rigorous standards as any medicine. They must be safe, effective and of reliable quality. Look for a nine number Product Licence (PL) number on the product container or packaging which is prefixed by the letters PL to see if a product is licensed.

If you buy herbal products over the Internet they may come from countries other than the UK, and could contain harmful herbs that are not permitted in the UK. Different countries have different regulations and some have none, so you are safest purchasing products that come from a known and regulated source.

History

Herbal medicine has been practised in the UK for tens of thousands of years. In the ancient world all civilisations used plants as natural remedies. Many plants contain chemicals that are of medicinal value, and some are used in modern medicine. Practitioners down the centuries have observed the effects of using different plants on different conditions and much of what is practised today is based on these traditional observations.

Key principles

A core principle behind herbal medicine is the idea that the whole plant offers a balanced benefit in a way that isolating a chemical from the plant does not. Some traditions believe that the physical appearance of a plant can determine what it should treat. Western herbalists are now more likely to use a herb for the chemicals contained within.

Different traditions

There are several branches of herbal medicine including:

- Western herbal medicine – with roots in Ancient Greece and Rome.
- The Ayurvedic tradition of India.
- Chinese herbal medicine.
- Traditional Tibetan medicine.

Most herbal medicine in the UK is offered on a private basis: you pay to consult a practitioner.

What is it used for?

Herbal medicine can be used to treat a wide range of conditions. You may have used echinacea to boost your immunity, ginger to help ease nausea or St John's wort when you are feeling depressed.

Dee Atkinson owns and runs Napiers the Herbalist in Edinburgh, one of the UK's oldest and best known herbal houses. Dee is also the director of NIMH, she explains, 'People consult us for all the same things as they would see a GP for. We tend to have more chronic complaints, simply because these tend to be management issues, and patients have realised that there is no "cure". Probably the main complaints are the menopause, irritable bowel syndrome, skin problems and arthritis.'

Herbal medicine works well for many different groups of people. The MHRA advises that the safety of many herbal medicines has not been established for:

- Pregnant women.
- Breastfeeding mothers.
- Children.
- Older people.

Problems can occur, for example, if you are pregnant or breastfeeding, as chemicals from herbal remedies can be transmitted through your bloodstream to your unborn baby or through breast milk.

If you come under one of these groups, or care for someone who does, be cautious when using herbal medicines and get advice from a practitioner rather than treating yourself. Herbalist Dee Atkinson advises, 'We run a parent and child clinic, and see a lot of pregnant women. I personally work with a lot of cancer patients. There are no barriers to who can be helped. We often work alongside the patient's GP or consultant.'

If you have a history of liver or kidney complaints, or any other serious health condition do not take any herbal medicine without speaking to your GP first. Herbal remedies can interact with other medicines, so if you take regular medication check with your GP then consult a registered herbalist.

Does it work?

There is evidence that specific herbal remedies or extracts of remedies are beneficial: herbs contain chemical compounds which have effects on the body. Medicines such as quinine and digitalis are well known for their plant origins. Dee Atkinson comments, 'Many of our plants contain constituents that have been synthesised into conventional drugs. Think of aspirin from willow bark, or the early contraceptive from wild yam. There is a lot of research on plants, and some herbs such as garlic, tumeric, devil's claw or St John's wort have become well known due to this. With many herbs there are thousands of years of use and knowledge of the plants.' Scientists looking to develop new medicines often use plant-based sources.

What's more, the tradition of herbal medicine means that a therapist will make up a specific combination of remedies, taking a holistic view on the person's overall health. Dee Atkinson explains, 'A herbalist will make a specific remedy for a person. We can sometimes use five herbs in a mix or we can use 15.' This personal approach makes it harder to evaluate using scientific research methods.

However many traditional remedies have not been subject to scientific studies, or such studies that have taken place have been small scale. More research needs to be done into herbal remedies in general.

How to find a practitioner

To help you select which herbal practitioner would suit you, consider:

- Suitability of their experience for your condition.
- Where they are located.
- Whether you'd prefer to be referred by a friend.
- The empathy between you and the practitioner.

If you are looking for a particular type of treatment, such as Chinese herbal medicine, you should check with the practice first that they offer that service.

If you plan to claim on private health insurance you will first need to check your level of cover, and whether you need to be referred by your GP or consultant, with your insurance company.

Choose a herbalist who is a member of a professional body that is within the EHTPA – look at their website for a list www.ehtpa.eu. See the help list for details of where you can find lists of herbal practitioners.

A typical treatment

You can expect your first herbal medicine appointment to take longer than subsequent appointments; it may last for an hour or more. The herbalist will ask you about your general health and your past history. Dee Atkinson explains, 'We do a full medical examination, take a medical history and ask a lot of questions about lifestyle and diet.' You may also be asked questions about:

- Your family's medical history.
- Your lifestyle.
- Your current complaint.
- Your medications.
- Any allergies you suffer from.

A herbalist may also do a physical examination, measure your blood pressure, check your pulse or take urine samples.

The practitioner will use all this information to diagnose your condition. They will make suggestions about how they could treat your condition with an individual prescription for herbal remedies plus possible changes to diet, exercise and lifestyle. If necessary, they will refer you on for other treatments which could include osteopathy, counselling, massage etc.

After the treatment

The herbalist will discuss with you any effects you may feel during and after the treatment. Follow-up consultations usually take place a few weeks after the initial appointment. These will be shorter, ranging from 20 to 30 minutes, depending on the treatment that you need. Your practitioner will ask you about any changes in your condition, and discuss how the treatment is progressing. They may adjust your remedies to take into account any changes. The number of sessions you need will depend on you and your health problem. Dee Atkinson explains, 'I have some patients who see me every three months just for a follow-up, some who see me every year, and others who I only see for two sessions. Chronic health care needs management, support and reassessment. We work with our patients on different levels, and some patients come back for counselling as much as for more medicine.'

Use with children

Some herbal remedies are considered to be safe to use with children and babies, but many do not have a proven safety record. When choosing a herbalist for a child, ask about their experience of working with children. You should remain with your child throughout the consultation process.

Use with pregnant women

Women are generally advised against using herbal medicine in pregnancy and labour: certainly speak to a practitioner rather than self-medicating. Any persistent symptoms should, however, still be reported to your midwife or GP.

When not to use herbal medicines

If you have an existing condition or are taking regular medication talk to your GP before using any sort of herbal remedy.

In the past some traditional remedies have used ingredients from endangered animals, these are now banned but you may want to check with your practitioner that they are not using animal products in your treatment. This should not discourage you from using herbal medicine, the vast majority of remedies are plant based and the new licensing scheme should ensure you can have confidence about what you are being treated with.

Chinese herbal medicine

Chinese herbal medicine dates back to the third century BC. It influences Western herbal medicine but has many differences too. It is a major part of regular health care provision in China, and now you are likely to find a practitioner on many UK high streets. You may find a Chinese herbal medicine practitioner is also an acupuncturist.

Chinese herbal medicine is used to treat a wide range of conditions and can include:

- Herbal remedies.
- Acupuncture.
- Dietary changes.
- Breathing and movement exercises, as in tai chi and qi gong.

It is based on the concepts of yin and yang. Practitioners look at the fundamental balance and harmony between the two and use the different techniques above to balance them.

In the UK you can find a Chinese herbal medicine practitioner through the Register of Chinese Herbal Medicine which represents over 450 fully qualified practitioners. www.rchm.co.uk.

Quick action checklist

■ Think about whether herbal medicine can help you and your particular condition.

■ Look for a herbalist and ask them about their experience of treating your condition.

■ Arrange an initial appointment if you feel herbal medicine could help you.

Summing Up

Herbal medicine is a safe and useful therapy for a wide range of conditions. It uses a holistic approach; this means that the practitioner looks at you as a whole person rather than simply treating a single part of you. You can buy herbal remedies over the counter or see a practitioner for individual diagnosis and treatment. Always opt for professional advice if you use any medication or have a health condition. Look out for a practitioner who is a member of a professional body as this offers you more protection should anything go wrong.

Chapter Five

Homeopathy

In homeopathy, diluted substances are given to the person, usually in tablet form, to trigger the body's natural healing system. A homeopath will prescribe the appropriate homeopathic remedy based on your symptoms. The principle of homeopathy is that 'like cures like'. If substances were given to us in large quantities they would see us producing symptoms similar to the problem trying to be cured yet smaller quantities that are diluted can encourage the body to heal itself by increasing natural energy levels.

Homeopathic remedies use extracts from animals and plants, minerals and salts. Parts of these substances are dissolved and diluted many times to form what homeopaths refer to as 'remedies'. The substances are diluted in either alcohol or water using a special technique. Remedies can contain a number of combinations of substances depending on the requirement of the individual. It is possible to use homeopathy alongside conventional medicine. The remedies used are non-toxic and therefore do not have side effects. Vegans and vegetarians should inform their practitioner if they do not wish to have a remedy that includes extracts from animals: a small number of extracts may include substances such as fur, poisons or milks.

Homeopathic remedies can be readily bought at pharmacies. However, these will not be tailored to your specific needs. A homeopath can work with you to devise a remedy made specifically to treat your individual case. Remedies are available in different potency scales referred to as the 'C scale'. The 6C potency is usually the one that you would use at home. Higher potencies should generally be left to qualified practitioners to use.

History

Homeopathy has been practised in the UK for around 200 years. It originates from Ancient Greece and the word 'homeopathy' comes from the Greek for 'similar disease'. In the late 18th century a German physician named Samuel Hahnemann was keen to explore alternative therapies. He took a particular interest in a practice using South American tree bark to treat malaria. Hahnemann took a dose of the bark on a daily basis and developed similar symptoms to somebody suffering with malaria. He concluded that for a drug to be effective it must produce symptoms that are similar to the disease that it is trying to treat.

A typical treatment

You can expect your first homeopathy appointment to take longer than subsequent appointments; it may last up to an hour and a half. The homeopath will want to take a detailed history about your general health and your past history. You may also be asked questions about your family's medical history and your general lifestyle.

Homeopaths take a holistic approach to working and will want to find out about your emotional state as well as your physical health. It is important that you answer honestly and keep an open mind during the consultation. You may be asked questions that you find surprising: for example you might be asked about your different preferences, such as whether you prefer the rain or the sunshine. This helps the practitioner to build up a thorough picture of you and will help to make a diagnosis and to find the best remedy to treat your condition.

All of the information that you provide will help the homeopath to decide what remedies would be best suited for you. You may be asked to take the remedy half an hour after eating and to avoid strong foods or drink. Some homeopaths will make a diagnosis at the first appointment; others may wish to see you at a follow-up appointment so that they can consider your case further. Ask at the time of booking what will happen and how many appointments you are likely to need.

Follow-up consultations usually take place a few weeks after the initial remedy has been given and can be expected to last around 30 minutes. Some health insurers cover the cost of homeopathic treatments. If you have a policy it is worth checking whether homeopathy is covered.

What is it used for?

Homeopathy can be used to treat a wide range of symptoms including:

- Skin complaints.
- Breathing difficulties.
- Depression.
- Allergies.
- Hormonal problems including menopausal symptoms.
- Tiredness and chronic fatigue.
- Iron and calcium deficiencies.

If you are considering using homeopathy, consult a homeopath to find out if they will be able to treat your symptoms effectively. Alternatively, there are now many books on the market that you can use to find out more about self-treating at home with homeopathy.

Contraindications

It is advisable for people with cancer and those on prescribed medication to discuss the use of homeopathy with their GP prior to seeking out treatment. The remedies used are natural and are considered to be very safe.

Use with children

Homeopathy is considered to be safe to use with children and babies. The remedies can be given in a sweet pill, powder or liquid meaning that it is easy to administer even to the very young. Many parents choose to add some homeopathic medicines to their first aid kit at home to help with minor health problems. Arnica is particularly helpful for bumps and bruises and can be bought in tablet form or as a cream. Chamomilla can give swift pain relief to babies who are teething and Calendula cream can help to soothe nappy rash.

Children tend to respond quickly to homeopathic treatments. A homeopath can treat a wide range of conditions, such as sleep disorders, digestive problems, emotional problems and menstrual problems in teenagers.

Karen Runacres is a homeopath and says, 'Children respond beautifully to homoeopathy. It can be used from birth and is ideal for colic and teething. Other childhood issues commonly treated include hay fever, allergies, eczema, asthma, first aid, fears and phobias, recurring ear, nose and throat problems and sleep issues.'

When choosing a homeopath for your child, ask about their experience of working with children. You should remain with your child throughout the consultation process.

Joanne tells us, 'My little boy was 5 years old when he was treated by a homeopath. He was such a worrier and spent a lot of time in tears. His teacher was forever calling me in to say that he'd been crying at school. He seemed to put an enormous amount of pressure on himself and then burst into tears if things weren't "just so". A friend of mine is a qualified homeopath and she told me that it can help with emotional issues. I decided that we had nothing to lose so gave it a try. I had to answer lots of questions about his health and wellbeing, she then prescribed a remedy. It was really easy to get him to take it as the tablets were tiny and sugar-coated. I did notice that he became a lot calmer and seemed happier within himself after a few weeks.'

Use with pregnant women

Many women use homeopathy in pregnancy and labour. Any persistent symptoms should, however, still be reported to your midwife or GP.

Homeopathy can be used to deal with a range of pregnancy symptoms including constipation, morning sickness and heartburn. The remedies are safe for both mother and baby as only small amounts of diluted natural substances are used.

Homeopathic remedies can also be used to help both during and after labour. A homeopath can recommend a labour kit to pack to see you throughout the delivery to the birth. Remedies can be prescribed for both physical and emotional symptoms.

Use with older people

The gentle nature of homeopathy makes it particularly suitable for older people. Always consult a GP if you're taking other medications and use homeopathy alongside conventional medicine rather than as an alternative.

Case study

Kirsty had suffered from a skin condition for a number of years, here she tells us about her experience of homeopathy.

'It first started when I was about 18 years old and I went on holiday with friends. My skin became covered in what I can only describe as like a nettle rash after exposure to the sun. It was incredibly painful and unsightly. On returning home I went to the GP and the only advice that I was given was to stay out of the sun. Each time I went on holiday the same thing happened and my skin erupted. Keeping out of the sun was not practical: even walking to the local shop could trigger the rash. I decided to visit a homeopath to see if they were able to prescribe anything for me.

'The first visit took around an hour and a half. I was a bit surprised by some of the questions to be honest. I expected it to be all about my medical history but she also covered my preferences for different things like the seasons and the weather. I had a follow-up consultation a week later where I was given a remedy. I admit to being sceptical as the pills were tiny. I took them as instructed letting them dissolve underneath my tongue. I had to avoid eating or having a drink for half an hour before. I was prescribed something called "Sol" which means sun. It was explained that I would be given a little of what was causing my symptoms. While the rash did not completely disappear I did find that it didn't flare up to the usual extent. Now I carry the remedy with me which I can buy over the counter and take it when we go on holiday.'

What the experts say

Homeopath Karen Runacres is based in the Worcester and Malvern area. Karen explains a little more about homeopathy, 'Homeopathy works on the whole person so a homeopath needs to understand all about you to create a picture of you as a whole. The belief is that your problem is one part of your whole body and may be affecting other parts of you without you realising it. Homeopathy identifies the susceptible area of your immune system and provides stimulus for the self healing to begin. Our susceptibilities are our weakness and they are individual. They are influenced by family genes, physical and emotional environments, diet and relaxation, habits and so on.

'Homeopathy can help with many conditions such as low energy, sleep problems, allergies, hormonal problems, anxiety and headaches to name but a few. It can be used with great effect alongside conventional medicine, although it is always advisable for the GP to be informed and treatment discussed. If you want to give homeopathy a try I would recommend contacting the Society of Homeopaths who keep a register of practitioners and can help you to find somebody in your local area. It is always reassuring to get a recommendation from someone who has already been treated by a homeopath too.'
Karen's details can be found in the help list or by contacting the Society of Homeopaths.

How to find a practitioner

The Society of Homeopaths has a list of practitioners who have met with their professional standard and practice in accordance with their ethics. The homeopaths listed also have full professional indemnity insurance. Those registered are able to use the initials RSHom after their names. You can log on to the website at www.homeopathy-soh.org.

Quick action checklist

- Visit a local health store or pharmacy to view the homeopathic remedies that they have in store to use at home.

- Take advice on using remedies at home.

- Consider visiting a homeopath for a remedy that is tailored to meet your individual needs.

Summing Up

Homeopathy is a holistic system of healing that is suitable for all and focuses on treating physical and emotional symptoms. The remedies used work with your body's own healing powers to promote wellbeing. Homeopathic remedies are gentle yet powerful. A remedy closest to your symptom will be prescribed to encourage your body's own healing process.

Chapter Six

Hypnotherapy

Hypnosis allows you to open your mind to suggestions so that you can make positive changes in your life. Hypnotherapy helps you to enter a deep state of relaxation, similar to being in a dream-like state. It can be used for a variety of reasons, including anxiety, stress management, personal development and to tackle phobias.

Virtually anybody can be hypnotised, although some people are easier to hypnotise than others. It is important that you find a therapist that you feel comfortable with as you need to be able to have trust and confidence in them so that you can relax fully. When you are hypnotised you remain in total control and if you want to come out of a hypnotic state for any reason you will be able to do so.

Sometimes people worry that they will lose control when they are hypnotised. Rest assured that when you are hypnotised you will be fully in control. You can even talk if you want to. It is impossible for a hypnotherapist to get you to do anything against your will. If you have seen a stage hypnotist perform you may be wondering how they therefore get people to take part in foolish acts – but remember all participants in stage hypnosis enter into the show voluntarily and are consenting to take part.

History

Throughout the centuries many cultures have used trance and therefore it is difficult to establish exactly when hypnotherapy began. It is thought that shamans and witch doctors were using hypnosis when they suspended their consciousness to reveal answers to questions that they had. Franz Mesmer, an Austrian physician, developed the theory of 'animal magnetism'. He claimed that disease occurred due to a blockage in the magnetic flow around the body. This magnetic flow is now sometimes referred to as 'life energy'. While releasing the blockages Mesmer would use what a hypnotherapist would now refer to as 'suggestion'. This is when the therapist uses certain words to suggest positive change.

James Braid first used the term 'hypnotism'. He was a Scottish surgeon who initially believed that hypnosis was simply trickery. He spent time conducting experiments and went on to become a supporter of hypnotism. Dr James Esdaile used hypnosis successfully during his time in India around the 1840s. He carried out thousands of operations using hypnotherapy, 19 of which were reported to be amputations.

A typical treatment

Your first session will take longer than subsequent sessions. The hypnotherapist will want to take a full history to assess your needs, this could take up to an hour and a half. This also allows you the opportunity to get to know your hypnotherapist better and to ask any questions that you may have. Sometimes it is useful to write questions down before the session so that you don't forget them. Depending on your issue you may only need one treatment but it is more common to have several sessions. Hypnotherapists try to help people in relatively few sessions and you will normally notice some changes by your third session.

After taking the information from you, the hypnotherapist should explain what they are about to do. Some therapists have a couch for you to lie on, others use a chair. Depending on the therapist you may be given headphones to wear and relaxing music might be played. You can expect the therapy room to be a clean and calming environment.

Everybody responds to hypnotherapy in a different way, but most people experience a feeling of deep relaxation. Your eyes are likely to feel heavy and close. You will be able to hear everything that is going on and you will be conscious of the therapist's voice. At times you may be unsure of what the hypnotherapist has said, but don't worry about this as it will be absorbed by your unconscious mind.

There are a number of ways that a hypnotherapist can induce a trance. Ask your hypnotherapist about the method that they use. Once you are in a trance the therapist will work on deepening the trance. You may be asked to imagine a pleasant place such as a garden or a beach. By deepening the sense of relaxation the hypnotherapist is able to access the subconscious mind more easily.

Your hypnotherapist may teach you self-hypnosis which is a simple method that you can use to relax at home. By using self-hypnosis you can strengthen suggestions that your therapist has made during the session. You may also be given a CD to listen to in-between sessions. Repeating a suggestion helps to strengthen it, which is why these methods are beneficial.

When your hypnotherapist brings you out of the trance you can expect to feel wide awake and energised. It is safe to drive home after a hypnotherapy session. You must not, however, drive or operate any machinery while listening to a hypnotherapy CD.

What is it used for?

Hypnotherapy can be used for a wide range of reasons including:

- Addictions.
- Relaxation.
- Phobias.
- Personal development, such as helping you to feel confident for public speaking.
- Changing behaviours, such as weight loss or smoking cessation.
- Pain control.
- Sexual disorders, such as erectile dysfunction, vaginismus and premature ejaculation.

Contraindications

Hypnotherapy should not be used if you have:

- Schizophrenia or personality disorders.
- Clinical depression, bipolar or other mental illness.
- Epilepsy or narcolepsy.
- Serious heart conditions.
- Dementia.

Use with children

Hypnotherapy can be used with children from around the age of 5 years old. Children can respond well to hypnotherapy. If you are considering using hypnotherapy for your child you should always ask the therapist about their experience in working with children. Children under the age of 16 years old should always be accompanied by a parent or guardian when receiving hypnosis. It can be particularly useful for dealing with anxieties, sleep difficulties, phobias and unwanted habits.

Jess tells us, 'My son is a worrier, he worries about everything. I wanted him to have some way of releasing his anxieties. I've tried hypnotherapy myself and found it very relaxing so decided to take him to see my therapist. She built up a great relationship with him and took the time to talk to him about the things that he is interested in. Based on this she developed a hypnotic script all about spaceships and rockets. Ben was able to fly to the moon and leave his worries there, he thought it was wonderful! I noticed that after a couple of sessions he became much calmer and less anxious in himself. We were given a CD that we use at home now from time to time.'

Use with pregnant women

Many pregnant women are now using hypnotherapy to aid the birth of their child. There has been much research into the area which suggests that hypnotherapy can be useful for reducing:

- The length of labour.

- The use of pain-controlling drugs during labour.

- The need for interventions, such as forceps or Caesarean deliveries.

It is recommended that women begin preparation for the birth with hypnotherapy at around 32 weeks. In the earlier stages of pregnancy women may wish to use hypnotherapy for relaxation purposes.

Charlotte tells us, 'I used a hypnotherapy CD in the run up to the birth of my last child. I listened to the CD every few days from around the time that I got to 35 weeks until the birth. I found the CD incredibly relaxing to listen to and often drifted off into a deep sleep. When I went into labour I listened to the CD a few times. I think that it did help me to relax which can only be a good thing. I can't say it shortened the labour or helped with the pain as I don't know how long I'd have been in labour if I'd not used it or how much pain I would have been in. This labour was, however, 10 hours shorter than my last labour! I'd recommend that pregnant women consider hypnotherapy even if it is just for the wonderful feeling of relaxation that they can gain.'

Use with older people

Older people can also benefit from hypnotherapy. If medication is being taken it is advisable to discuss the use of hypnotherapy first with your GP.

Case studies

Often people can be sceptical about hypnotherapy, here John tells us about his experience.

'I was extremely sceptical about trying hypnotherapy but after suffering with a fear of flying for years I decided it was worth a go. The therapist was extremely professional and took time to put me at ease. My only experience of hypnotherapy had been what I had seen on the stage, yet this experience was nothing at all like that. I felt calm and in control. After just one session I felt much less anxious about flying. On our next family holiday I was able to board the plane without feeling any fear. Usually I would head straight to the bar and have several drinks in the departure lounge to calm my nerves but I didn't feel the need to do this at all. I was given a CD to use at home if I felt I needed it. I've not used it as my anxiety levels have remained low, it is reassuring though to know I have it if I need to use it in the future.'

Sally wanted to give up smoking and turned to hypnotherapy.

'I really didn't think that it would work, even while I was being hypnotised I felt doubtful. I was proved wrong however and hypnotherapy gave me the strength to stop smoking, I couldn't believe it.'

What the experts say

Lynn Wilshaw is a qualified and experienced hypnotherapist. As well as running a practice from her office in South Yorkshire, Lynn also has an online store selling hypnotherapy CDs for use at home. To view the CDs visit Lynn's website at www.hippohypno.co.uk.

Lynn tells us, 'Hypnotherapy helps people to live the life they want to live. It equips them to be able to handle day-to-day stresses, they can become more able to take control of their lives and to move forward in a positive way.

'I always try to remember that it is not easy to talk to a stranger about difficulties that they are experiencing. I personally try to make the person feel comfortable and at ease. I undertake an initial assessment procedure to see what they wish to achieve from the therapy and if this is realistic. If it is, then I can usually give them an idea of how many sessions may be required. I then always give them the option to go away and think about it. I don't want to pressurise people into making an appointment, I want them to feel that I am the right therapist for them and I want to offer them a professional service that they value. Finding the right hypnotherapist for you is important if the treatment is going to be a success.'

How to find a practitioner

Find a hypnotherapist who is a member of the Hypnotherapy Society by logging on to the website at www.hypnotherapysociety.com. Further contact details for the society can be found in the useful contacts section at the back of this book. You may also wish to check whether there are any local therapists registered with the General Hypnotherapy Register, which is the largest professional register of therapists in the UK at www.general-hypnotherapy-register.com.

Josephine Teague from the Cambridge College of Hypnotherapy reminds us, 'It is vital that you feel comfortable with the therapist. Research has shown that it is the interaction of client and therapist that allows the changes to happen. This is probably the most important point of all. Always work with a therapist that you feel you can trust and you are comfortable with.'

Quick action checklist

- Consider purchasing a hypnotherapy CD to use at home.
- Find out about local hypnotherapists and check that they are registered with an appropriate professional body.
- Book an initial appointment with a hypnotherapist to discuss your requirements.

Summing Up

Hypnotherapy is a complementary therapy that can be useful for dealing with a wide range of difficulties. If you think that it is something that you may like to try, spend some time researching local therapists. Some therapists specialise in certain areas, such as weight loss, phobias or working with children.

Chapter Seven

Massage

Massage is a method of manipulating the layers of muscle and connective tissues to enhance their functioning and promote relaxation. Friction improves the circulation of blood and enables the release of toxins. It also stimulates and relaxes the muscles, reduces or eliminates pain, lowers blood pressure and heartbeat and allows deep relaxation to occur. The body is manipulated manually and specific areas can be targeted. A therapist will usually apply pressure with their hands or fingers, although they can also use their elbows, knees or even their feet.

There are many different types of massage, including sports massage, Indian head massage and Swedish massage. A full body massage will work on each muscle group of the body. An Indian head massage will concentrate on the back, neck, arms, head and face. This can be useful for helping to relieve headaches, sinusitis and reducing tension in the shoulders. A sports therapy massage can help to restore pain-free movement to ligaments and joints. It is often the non-sportsperson who can benefit most from these types of massage, so don't be put off by the name.

Many therapists offer a range of massage services, so if you are unsure about which type of massage will suit your needs best, you should discuss it prior to making an appointment.

Most massage is given using oil, such as sunflower, almond or coconut. This makes the friction smooth and comfortable. These carrier oils also have therapeutic effects. Some therapists add aromatherapy oils and occasionally salts can be used in association with oils in order to remove any hard skin.

History

Massage is thought to date back to ancient times and was used by the Romans and Egyptians. The Greek physicians put great emphasis on the benefits of massage. Hippocrates instructed physicians on the benefits of rubbing during the fifth century BC. In Romania a tame bear was used to tread on patients in order to massage them to cure them of disease. There has always been an awareness of the healing nature of massage and if we are hurt we instinctively reach to rub it better. The benefits of massage were documented in the West, although few advances were made until the 19th century. In the 1800s Per Henrik Ling introduced a system of massage to treat physical issues, which included techniques such as stroking, pressing and squeezing. His system became known as Swedish Massage and is the basis of many Western massage techniques. In the East, massage has been used for even longer than has been documented in the West.

Massage was used during World War 1 to treat those who suffered from shell shock. During the 1960s people became interested in massage, not only for its physical benefits, but also as a way of dealing with stress. As a result massage has become a respected form of complementary therapy. Today, a multitude of massage techniques are practised to help to promote physical and emotional wellbeing.

A typical treatment

There are many different types of massage treatment available and massage can be used to treat many different parts of the body, together or individually, from full body massages to neck and back massages, Indian head massage to foot massage. In order to find out exactly what the treatment will involve you should speak to the therapist at the time of booking.

You can generally expect a massage to take from 30 minutes to an hour and a half, depending on the treatment you choose. Your first appointment may take longer as the therapist will want to discuss your medical history and what you are hoping to gain from the session. The room that is used should be quiet and clean. You will be asked to either sit on a special chair or lie on a couch, depending on the type of massage that you are to receive.

Clothing will usually have to be removed for massage to take place. If this is necessary the therapist will leave the room while you undress to your underwear and provide you with blankets or towels so that you can cover yourself up. The therapist will keep the parts of the body that they are not working on covered up. Some massage treatments can be performed fully clothed, although you should take care to wear loose and comfortable clothing.

Relaxing music may be played and the lights are often dimmed. You may wish to close your eyes to aid your relaxation. If there is a particular area that you do not want to be massaged do tell the therapist. For example, some people don't like their feet to be touched. Or if there is an area of your body that you would like special attention to be paid to, make sure that you let them know.

The therapist will work on your body and should check to see that you are comfortable with the amount of pressure that they are applying. It is important that you should tell the practitioner if you are uncomfortable with any part of the treatment. Once the massage is completed you will be asked to get dressed in your own time and usually be given a drink of water.

What is it used for?

Massage can be used for a variety of purposes including:

- Pain relief, particularly from back and neck pain.
- The reduction of stress and anxiety.
- Improving the comfort and fluidity of movement generally.
- Removing toxicity from the body.
- Improving digestion and the functioning of all the organs in the body.
- To increase energy.
- For relaxation.
- Insomnia.
- Stimulating the immune system.
- To improve circulation.

Contraindications

Massage should not be used in certain circumstances. These include:

- If you have deep vein thrombosis.
- When there are any bleeding disorders or warfarin is being taken.
- If blood vessels are seriously damaged.
- If you have a fracture.
- Where bones are weakened through cancer or osteoporosis.
- If you have a fever.

Always discuss your medical history with your practitioner prior to treatment taking place and seek the advice of your GP if you are in any doubt as to whether massage is suitable for you.

Use with children

Babies in particular can benefit from massage and it can be relaxing for both the child and the parent. Massage can help to encourage better sleeping, relieve colic and may help to boost the youngster's immune system. Aromatherapy oils should not be used and nut oils should also be avoided. Sunflower oil works well for massage. Specialist classes are available for parents to learn massage skills, ask your health visitor to find out if any are running in your area. The International Association of Infant Massage can also provide you with details of local practitioners and classes if you visit their website at www.iaim.org.uk.

Rachel tells us, 'I used massage with all three of my children. I found that the best time was after their bath before I got them ready for bed. It helped us to bond and I regarded it as our "special" time. I think all three of them found it really relaxing and I'm sure that it helped them to sleep. I really enjoyed performing baby massage too and I found it a relaxing time. I went to a class at my local children's centre. The course was only £1.50 each week for four weeks and the bonus was that I got to meet other new mums in my area too.'

Use with pregnant women

There are a number of practitioners who now specialise in offering massage to pregnant women. It is important that the therapist is experienced in working with pregnant women. You should lie in a semi-reclined position and extra cushions should be used to ensure that you are supported and comfortable while you are on your side.

If you are at risk of premature labour or have other pregnancy-related difficulties you should consult your midwife before massage takes place and also inform your therapist.

Suzi says, 'I had a massage when I was around six months pregnant and it was wonderful! I had a particularly difficult pregnancy and was large right from the beginning. Everything seemed to ache, my feet, legs, back, you name it! I was a bit worried about having a massage in case it did any damage to our baby, but I researched it thoroughly and found a practitioner who specialises in this area. It was probably the most wonderful hour of my pregnancy, all the aches and pains that I had melted away and I felt completely relaxed. Later on in the pregnancy I suffered badly with swollen feet. I turned to massage again and it really helped with the discomfort. Now I've had the baby I'm continuing to have massages on a regular basis as I find them incredibly relaxing and helpful with any back pain that I may have.'

Use with older people

Elderly people can also benefit from massage. If you're elderly, you may have undiagnosed pain in your joints. It is important that massage takes place just above or below these areas to improve circulation. As the body is older it may require gentler techniques to be used. If you use a wheelchair it is possible to receive massage while in the chair. Time is usually spent on hands and feet to improve circulation. Human touch can be a real pleasure for the young and old alike.

Case study

Robert enjoys a massage on a regular basis after receiving his first as a birthday treat last year.

'I'd never really considered going for a massage before. I thought it was just for women to be honest. Somebody bought me a gift voucher for a massage and I went along to see what it was like. I have a full body massage now on a regular basis and really look forward to these sessions.

'The actual massage lasts for about an hour. There are different types that you can have and they last varying amounts of time. My therapist uses aromatherapy oils too when massaging me and chooses masculine scents, I was a bit worried at first that I'd smell very feminine! I strip down to my boxer shorts but remain covered underneath a blanket. The therapist just moves the blanket aside to massage the area that she is working on. I often fall asleep while being massaged, I find the whole experience incredibly relaxing. I make sure that I have nothing planned after an appointment now as I like to just go home and enjoy the feeling of calm that washes over me. I really wish that I'd tried massage sooner, it helps me unwind in a way that I've not experienced before.'

What the experts say

Marion Eaton is an experienced therapist from Hastings who is trained in Swedish massage, holistic massage, professional aromatherapy, and NO HANDS Massage® as well as other forms of bodywork. She advises, 'When deciding what type of massage you should book, you can begin by considering what sort of touch you like. If, for example, you like a deep massage then you may want to opt for a sports massage or lymphatic drainage. If you prefer a more soothing touch you could consider an aromatherapy massage or maybe a facial massage. Sometimes you need to take into account practical considerations. For example, Thai massage involves you lying on a futon on the floor – if you have mobility problems this may not be possible.'

Marion points out the importance of the environment where the massage takes place, 'Having a massage is a multi-sensory experience which can involve soft lighting, calming music, scents and touch. The environment that the massage is carried out in is therefore very important and you should consider this when booking a session.

'I generally recommend that people attend for weekly massages for the first six weeks. You should then review this with your practitioner in order to decide what will best meet your needs. I believe that people can benefit from massage in every single way, physically, mentally and emotionally. Massage benefits all organs of the body, relaxes muscles and helps blood to flow. Emotionally it acts as a great release and helps you to relax. When you book a massage, you make a gift of time to yourself. It is very important to recognise that you deserve that time and treatment to keep you well, and to promote and maintain your wellbeing.'

To find out more about Marion's work log on to her website at www.marioneaton.com and to find out more about her work with NO HANDS® Massage visit www.marioneaton.org.uk.

Rakhee Shah carries out a number of different types of massage. Here she tells us about Indian head massage and what you can expect, 'An Indian head massage can take between 30-45 minutes and is usually performed with the client being seated. I ask my clients to try to relax and to place their hands on their legs and close their eyes. I begin by rocking the head backwards and forwards to loosen the muscles in the neck and relax the client. Both sides of the neck are then massaged in an upwards circular motion. Next the shoulder area is massaged using various strokes. Along with the shoulder area, the rest of the upper back is massaged as well as the spine area followed by the arms. Then comes what I consider to be the really pleasurable part, the head and face massage. First the head is massaged starting with the back of the head, various massage techniques are applied. The face is then massaged, beginning with the forehead, massaging around the eyes, sinus areas, mouth to ear and finally the chin. The client is then balanced so that all negative energy is dispersed of and positive energy is given.'

Rakhee goes on to explain the benefits of Indian head massage, 'It is good for relaxation and can help people who suffer from stress, headaches, loss of hair or insomnia. It is advisable to have one treatment and to see how you feel.

Some people do get side effects such as headaches, dizziness, tiredness, sickness but this can be a good sign indicating that the body is releasing negative energies. Check with your therapist about the contraindications, these include things like a high temperature, skin infections, head, shoulder or neck injury and epilepsy. Generally however, Indian massage is one of the safest treatments available.' Rakhee is based in New Barnet, Hertfordshire. To find out more log on to her site at www.haveamassage.co.uk.

How to find a practitioner

Massage Therapy UK provides information about massage and has a directory of practitioners that can be searched online at www.massagetherapy. co.uk. The General Council for Massage Therapies is the governing body for massage therapists in the UK. They can also help you to find a practitioner by visiting their website at www.gcmt.org.uk.

Quick action checklist

- Consider the different types of massage available and which one would be most appropriate to meet your needs.
- Purchase some massage oil to use at home. It is readily available from health stores.
- Research local therapists and what types of massage they offer.

Summing Up

Touch is a very powerful force that can help to ease pain, release tension, soothe emotions and promote relaxation. You will feel the benefits long after the massage is finished and be able to function more efficiently. In today's fast-paced life we often forget to take time out to care for ourselves, massage can help to redress the balance. Massage is not just relaxing, it is also revitalising and can leave you feeling rejuvenated.

Massage can be performed virtually anywhere, making it a very flexible treatment. It is becoming increasingly common for therapists to visit the workplace as managers recognise that investing in their employees' wellbeing can be a rewarding experience for the company. There are now numerous instructional books and DVDs on the market if you would like to learn some basic massage skills and many local colleges offer short courses to teach you the basics.

Chapter Eight

Osteopathy

In osteopathy practitioners treat your muscles and bones and can work with your organs, ligaments, cartilage, fibrous tissue, blood vessels, nerves and glands. It uses a holistic approach: this means that the osteopath looks at you as a whole person rather than simply treating a single part of you.

Osteopaths are skilled in using manual and physical techniques to treat and sometimes prevent health problems. Most commonly, osteopathy is used for back and neck pain. Osteopaths are taught that treating the bones, muscles and joints encourages your body to heal.

An osteopath will assess your general and physical health before checking the way that you stand and how different parts of your body move. An osteopath can work with you over a period of months, weeks or days to treat pain and movement problems and help your health and wellbeing.

Regulation and safety

The General Osteopathic Council (GOsC) regulates the practice of osteopathy in the UK. By law osteopaths must be registered with the GOsC in order to practise in the UK. Osteopath Jane Jeater (www.janejeater.co.uk) explains, 'To achieve registration, osteopaths have to attend a registered college and graduate with a four or five year bachelor degree in osteopathy.'

Only those registered can use the title 'osteopath'. The GOsC sets, maintains and develops standards of osteopathic practice and conduct. Osteopaths have to re-register each year after completing a set standard of training, known as continued professional development. All osteopaths are expected to have a complaints procedure and would be happy to discuss your concerns. If you are unable to resolve the issue with the osteopath, you can contact the GosC for advice.

Key principles

According to the British School of Osteopathy, a core principle behind osteopathy is the idea that 'the body is an integrated and indivisible whole, and contains self-healing mechanisms that can be utilised as part of the treatment'. This means that the osteopath will ask you about relevant psychological and social factors as well as your physical health.

The aim of osteopathic treatment is:

- Understanding what is wrong.
- Pain relief and management.
- Increased mobility.
- Strategies and advice for reducing the likelihood of the problem reoccurring.
- Return to work, sport, and everyday activities.
- Improved health and wellbeing.

History

Osteopathy has been practised in the UK for around a hundred years. The therapy began in the US in 1874 where it was named 'osteopathy' by Andrew Taylor Still of Kansas, who founded the American School of Osteopathy. He called the therapy 'osteopathy' as he felt that 'the bone, osteon, was the starting point from which [he] was to ascertain the cause of pathological conditions. In the US osteopaths are known as Doctors of Osteopathy, which is a medical qualification.

Osteopathy is now practised across Europe, Israel, Canada, New Zealand and Australia, South Africa and Zimbabwe. In 1917 John Martin Littlejohn founded the first UK osteopathic college, the British School of Osteopathy. Littlejohn had studied under Andrew Taylor Still, but added in the study of physiology to his training programme. Osteopaths in the UK are not generally doctors. A small number of doctors undertake osteopathic training.

Most osteopathy in the UK is offered on a private basis. A small number of general practices choose to fund an osteopath to provide treatment on the NHS.

What is it used for?

Osteopathy can be used to treat a wide range of conditions. Osteopath Lin Bridgeford (www.osteo-info.co.uk) says, 'My practice is very broad. Back and neck problems are very common, also all other joints – hips, knees, ankles, feet, wrists, hands, elbows and shoulders. I treat people with post trauma and whiplash injuries, and offer pre- and post-operative help.'

Osteopathy is best known for treating back and neck problems, but can also help:

- Arthritis and spondylitis.
- Back pain.
- Carpal tunnel syndrome.
- Changes to posture during pregnancy.
- Foot pain.
- Frozen shoulder.
- General stiffness and tension.
- Headaches.
- Joint pain.
- Neck pain.
- Pelvic, hip and leg pain.
- Repetitive strain injuries.
- Sciatica or trapped nerves.
- Shoulder and arm pain.
- Minor sports injuries.
- Work injuries.
- Symptoms of stress.

Osteopathy works well for many different groups of people. Jane Jeater comments, 'Osteopathy is suitable for anyone from babies and children, sports people, manual workers, office workers and older people. Osteopathy is also safe during pregnancy.' Groups that find osteopathy helpful include:

- Mothers-to-be during pregnancy.

- Babies – see cranial osteopathy in particular.

- Children and teenagers.

- People with sports injuries.

- People with driving or work-related problems.

- Older people.

If you are considering using osteopathy for a particular condition, ask the osteopath if they are able to treat your condition effectively.

Does it work?

There is growing evidence that osteopathy is beneficial for lower back pain and other conditions. Jane Jeater explains, 'In 2004, the Medical Research Council found spinal manipulation, added to GP care, is clinically effective for back pain. In 2006 the Department of Health published guidelines that recognised that osteopathy can quickly and effectively resolve musculoskeletal disorders, and in 2009 The National Institute for Health and Clinical Excellence published guidelines that recommended manual therapy, such as osteopathy for non-specific lower back pain. In addition there is ongoing research on a variety of aspects of osteopathy'.

A 2005 review of six trials of osteopathic manipulative treatment concluded that it significantly reduces lower back pain (Licciardone et al., 2005). And several large studies in the UK have shown positive clinical and cost-effectiveness of manipulation in the management of lower back pain, the latest being the UK Back Pain Exercise and Manipulation (UK BEAM) trial.

How to find a practitioner

Osteopath Jane Jeater explains, 'You don't need a GP's referral to see an osteopath. However many GPs do refer their patients to osteopaths. It is easy to get an appointment. The GOsC state that 54% of new patients are seen within one working day, and 95% are seen within one week. Many major private health insurance policies provide cover for osteopathic treatment – check with your own provider before booking.'

Contact the General Osteopathic Council, www.osteopathy.org.uk, to find a practitioner. All osteopaths are registered with this governing body. Osteopath Jane Jeater advises, 'By law all osteopaths must be registered with the General Osteopathic Council. You can search the UK statutory register at www.osteopathy.org.uk/information/finding-an-osteopath. Many osteopaths are also members of the British Osteopathic Association, who have a members' directory on their website, www.osteopathy.org. Some osteopaths have a special interest or field they work in and there are organisations that represent them. Visceral osteopaths and those interested in sports are listed at www.osca.org.uk. There are also a small number of osteopaths who treat animals. They are represented by The Society of Osteopaths in Animal Practice.'

To help you select which osteopath would suit you, consider:

- Suitability of their experience.
- Whether you want an osteopath with a specialty.
- Where they are located.
- Whether you'd prefer to be referred by a friend.
- The empathy between you and the osteopath.
- Would you prefer a male or female osteopath.

If you are looking for a particular type of treatment, such as cranial osteopathy, you should check with the practice first that they offer that service.

If you plan to claim on private health insurance you will first need to check your level of cover, and whether you need to be referred by your GP or consultant, with your insurance company. You also need to check if the osteopath is registered with your insurance company.

A typical treatment

You can expect your first osteopathy appointment to take longer than subsequent appointments; it may last for an hour. You may need to check if the osteopath is registered. The osteopath will ask you about your general health and your past history. You may also be asked questions about your family's medical history and your general lifestyle. The osteopath will need to see how you move, so wear comfortable and non-restrictive clothes and be prepared to take off outer garments.

Then the osteopath will assess you physically by:

■ Examining your muscles and joints.

■ Observing your movements.

■ Moving some of your joints.

Depending on your particular problems, your osteopath may arrange for you to have X-rays, scans or other clinical investigation.

Once the osteopath has a clear idea of your health, they will discuss your treatment options. Jane Jeater advises, 'The osteopath will devise a treatment plan, and estimate how many treatments you should need. The number of treatments needed will depend on how long you have had the problem, the severity of the problem, and whether there are any ongoing medical, occupational or lifestyle factors that are contributing to, or maintaining the problem.' Typically osteopaths use gentle, non-invasive manual techniques, such as deep tissue massage, joint articulation and manipulation.

Osteopath Mark Pitcairn-Knowles says, 'A common misconception is that osteopathic treatment is rough. This is not true; they will occasionally apply a sharp thrust to a joint that may create a small "crack" sound. This is done to help reduce muscle tightness, but the osteopath will always ask for consent and ensure that there is no pain or discomfort as this would be counterproductive. Most treatment will consist of soft tissue massage, joint stretching, sports technique advice, exercise prescription and lifestyle corrections.' Your osteopath may also make suggestions about posture and diet, or refer you on to a different practitioner if necessary.

After the treatment

The osteopath will discuss with you any side effects you may feel during and after the treatment. Jane Jeater advises, 'Some techniques can cause discomfort. You must let your osteopath know if you are in pain or discomfort so they can modify the treatment to suit you. Patients occasionally report feeling tired, stiff and achy for the first 24 hours after treatment.'

Follow-up consultations usually take place a week after the initial appointment. These will be shorter, ranging from 20 minutes to 45 minutes depending on the treatment that you need. Your osteopath will ask you about any changes in your condition, carry out a reassessment of your muscles, joints and movements and then treat you.

Osteopath Mark Pitcairn-Knowles often sees people with sports-related injuries in his clinic (www.SpringbankClinic.co.uk). He explains, 'Osteopaths will apply the principles of osteopathy to sports injuries in the same way in which they approach other complaints. In a "sports injury" it is the manner of the injury that is different as well as the needs of the patient, both psychological and physical. The main osteopathic principle is that "structure governs function".'

Osteopathy for sports injuries

An osteopath deals with simple muscle damage by using soft tissue massage and stretching techniques. It is important to understand why the injury occurred in the first place so as to prevent it happening again. This could be:

- Trauma, like being trodden on.

- Stress and fatigue in the person's life.

- Poor technique, for example too much upper body pivot in rowing strains the lower back.

- Being overweight or lacking strength so levels of activity need to be sensibly planned.

Joints that are close to the muscle damage need to be assessed. If they work well the osteopath will look at how the body works further from the site. We all have individual shapes; the key things the osteopath will look for is how the shape works, are the joints supported by muscle and is there anything that can be done to improve or control the function.

Joint pain can be due to various tissues being damaged, such as bone, ligament, fascia, cartilage, or nerve. Osteopaths are good at identifying how a joint functions, asking themselves questions like:

- What is the range of movement?
- What is the quality of the movement like, stiff or loose?

They can improve joint range of movement, by manually stretching the joints and showing exercises for the person to do at home. If joint pain is due to the joint being too loose, then the osteopath will prescribe muscle-strengthening exercises. They will also look at whether injuries elsewhere have caused loss of movement in other joints that result in strain on the mobile area. These injuries are often due to repetitive activities rather than one-off traumas; hence an understanding of sport technique is important. Examples of this include a cyclist who may have stiffness in their upper back from an old car crash or simply working at a desk for long hours but as a result of reaching down to the handle bars while looking up with their head will develop neck pain and headaches. A horse rider with an arthritic hip will compensate for the lack of movement in the hip and will try to sit correctly by arching their lower back.

When not to use osteopathy

It is advisable not to use osteopathy on a fractured bone and practitioners may be able to offer limited help if you suffer from osteoporosis. Mark Pitcairn-Knowles explains, 'Osteopaths pride themselves on their ability to diagnose where a condition is not suitable for osteopathic treatment and can refer to a suitable destination for more appropriate treatment.'

You may be advised against using osteopathy if you have cancer or blood-clotting problems: practitioners advise that gentle cranial treatment can be beneficial and safe in these cases. If you have health conditions, discuss the use of osteopathy with your GP before to seeking out treatment. Always discuss your medical history with your osteopath prior to treatment taking place. Osteopath Lin Bridgeford explains, 'Osteopaths are trained to recognise and treat a wide range of conditions, when not to treat and when to refer to a doctor. The GOsC logo includes the words "Safe in our hands".' She continues, 'There are many techniques that can be adapted to each person or situation. Some techniques would be unsuitable for some people, for example manipulation with the use of high velocity thrust would not be used on babies or someone with osteoporosis; some conditions would require an X-ray or MRI before treating. This can be determined during the initial consultation.'

Use with children

Osteopathy is considered to be safe to use with children and babies. When choosing an osteopath for your child, ask about their experience of working with children. You should remain with your child throughout the consultation process.

Use with pregnant women

Many women use osteopathy in pregnancy. Any persistent symptoms should, however, still be reported to your midwife or GP. Osteopathy can be used to deal with a range of physical pregnancy symptoms.

Cranial osteopathy

Cranial osteopathy was created after Dr William Sutherland observed that it is possible to make microscopic movements of the bone plates that make up the skull. It can help with a range of conditions. There is less research into the therapy than into osteopathy. One study has indicated that it can help babies with colic but more research is needed. It is used to help with:

Trauma after a difficult birth.

Plagiocephaly (misshapen head).

Newborn irritability and restlessness.

Crying babies.

Colic, sickness and wind.

Feeding difficulties.

Sleep disturbances.

Ear infections.

Sinus and adenoidal problems.

Headaches.

Behaviour problems.

Childhood injuries.

Cranial osteopaths can be found at www.sutherlandcranialcollege.co.uk/aboutus/memberslist/.

Case study

Nell has used osteopathy during and after pregnancy. She says, 'With my first pregnancy I had a lot of back pain. I was fortunate that my GP's surgery had an osteopath in every day, so I was referred to see him. It helped enormously. I had a session every week or so, which continued after I had given birth until I felt that my back had recovered and I stopped getting pain. With my most recent pregnancy I experienced pelvic girdle pain. The relaxing hormones released during pregnancy meant that the two halves of my pelvis could click out of alignment and the osteopath really helped by gently realigning me every week or two. This time, having moved house, I paid around £30 for each session. It was worth the money, though, as it was the only thing that helped.'

Quick action checklist

- Think about whether osteopathy can help you and your particular condition.
- Look for an osteopath and ask them about their experience of treating your condition.
- Arrange an initial appointment if you feel osteopathy could help you.

Summing Up

Osteopathy is a safe and useful therapy for a wide range of conditions. It uses a holistic approach: this means that the osteopath looks at you as a whole person rather than simply treating a single part of you.

Osteopaths are trained to use manual and physical techniques to treat and sometimes prevent health problems. Most commonly, osteopathy is used for back and neck pain: research has proved it is effective for lower back pain.

There are osteopaths across the UK; find one that has experience in treating your condition. You will find the treatment involves a mix of gentle, non-invasive manual techniques, such as deep tissue massage and joint articulation and manipulation. You may feel stiff or achy initially after your treatment but should see a gradual improvement. You may need to see an osteopath for several sessions, and some people consult on an ongoing basis to keep pain or conditions under control.

Chapter Nine

Reiki

Reiki pronounced 'ray key' is a natural system of healing. Many reiki practitioners and teachers believe that this universal life force energy is, quite simply, the power of unconditional love. Although reiki's roots are in Buddhist qigong, it is not part of any religious belief system. Anyone can learn to give reiki if their intention is pure, and anyone or anything can receive it.

The Eastern tradition that gave birth to reiki teaches that we are multi-dimensional beings, not merely a physical body. To be truly healthy all parts of our being, body, mind, emotions and spirit need to be clear and in balance. The pressures of modern living are constantly causing imbalances in our personal energy ('qi') and so we often feel low and depleted. It is in this state that our immune system comes under severe stress. This stress will manifest on some level of our being, possibly as physical pain or sickness, but often as mental illness such as depression, or emotional problems like fear or anxiety.

The reiki practitioner acts as a bridge or transformer to reconnect the recipient to the universal life energy by channelling the reiki energy through their hands. The hands are usually placed gently on the body in hand positions which may correspond to the seven major chakras of the body (energy centres found in various areas of your body). However, experienced reiki practitioners often work intuitively and allow their hands to be drawn to those parts of the body which require healing. The touch is generally light and soothing; sometimes the treatment is performed without physical touch – the hands are held slightly above the body.

There are three levels of training to become a reiki master. These are referred to as the first, second and master degrees. At each of these degrees the student receives 'attunements' to the reiki energy from their reiki master teacher. These attunements gradually bring the higher vibrations of the reiki energy into the energy field of the student.

At first degree level a student learns to use reiki to heal themselves and others. The emphasis is on physical healing. At second degree level they are taught 'keys' or 'symbols' to enable them to heal on the emotional and mental levels. They also learn 'distance healing'. This means that they are able to treat others who are geographically located at a distance. At this point many students take an advanced reiki training to learn more techniques and to further build up the amount of reiki energy they can channel. A practitioner who is qualified to master level takes responsibility for their own healing and learns to help others deal with soul issues. They also learn to pass attunements to teach or 'attune' others to reiki.

Reiki can be used for many purposes, including healing animals, places and situations.

History

Hands on healing has been around for many thousands of years and used by different cultures. The history of reiki is constantly being rewritten as more and more information comes to light from Japan. What we do know is that Dr Mikao Usui discovered reiki in 1922 while on a 21-day retreat on Mount Kurama. In his lifetime Dr Usui taught over 2,000 students. He adopted and adapted a set of principles originally set down by a wise emperor of Japan which later became known as the Five Reiki Precepts:

At least for today:

- Do not be angry.

- Do not worry.

- Be grateful.

- Work with diligence.

- Be kind to people.

After Usui's death, one of the reiki masters that he trained, Dr Chujiro Hayashi, continued to spread reiki, as did several other of Dr Usui's disciples. Dr Hayashi developed the healing system introducing more hand positions and altering the attunement process. By the time of his death he had trained 14 reiki masters, including Mrs Takata. It was Mrs Takata who is credited with bringing reiki to the West and by her death in 1980 she had attuned 22 reiki masters. Reiki is now one of the fastest growing complementary therapies being taught. Each reiki practitioner can trace their reiki lineage back to Dr Mikao Usui.

A typical treatment

The first treatment may take longer as your practitioner takes time to get to know you and to find out what you hope to achieve through the sessions. Appointments generally last from 45 minutes to an hour and a half.

You will be asked to lie down on a couch and will remain fully clothed throughout, although you may remove your shoes. You should choose to wear loose and comfortable clothing so that you can relax. The atmosphere will be calming and sometimes soothing music is used, lights are dimmed and candles lit. Some practitioners will provide a home-visit service if this is more convenient for you.

The practitioner may spend a few minutes quietly preparing for your treatment before they begin by placing their hands over different parts of your body. Some practitioners may place their hands lightly onto your body, others may allow their hands to hover a few centimetres above the body, never making physical contact. Some practitioners will use a set sequence of hand movements, others will work more freely placing their hands where they feel the reiki is most needed. What you experience will vary from person to person. Some people report feeling warmth or tingling sensations, others report feeling incredibly well and relaxed. Reiki will flow to you in the correct quantity needed. It is advisable to drink water following a treatment.

What is it used for?

Reiki can be used for a variety of purposes including:

- Pain relief.
- Emotional release.
- Relaxation.

- Stress relief.
- To boost energy levels.
- To promote the body's ability to heal itself.
- To aid sleep.

Contraindications

Reiki is a very safe system of healing. You should not use reiki as a substitute for medical advice and, even if you feel your problem has been resolved, should always seek your GP's advice before stopping medication. Make sure that you discuss any medical problems with the reiki practitioner prior to treatment so that they can be fully aware of your needs.

Use with children

Children can enjoy receiving reiki. Some parents report that their child's behaviour has calmed as a result. If you are interested in trying reiki with your child, ask the practitioner what experience they have of working with children and confirm that you will be able to accompany your child throughout the treatment.

Sarah says, 'I first used reiki with my son when he was four years old. He used to be constantly on the go and found it difficult to settle to sleep. I'm a reiki master and thought I would give it a go and see what the results were. I found that if he came for a cuddle and I started to use reiki that he would settle for longer. He commented on Mummy's warm hands; when I use reiki my hands do become very hot to the touch. I saw a decrease in his hyperactive behaviour and attribute this to using reiki.'

Use with pregnant women

Reiki can be used throughout pregnancy and can help to relieve some of the stress that the mum-to-be may be feeling. Reiki can also be used during labour and a new trend is to 'attune' fathers so that they can treat their partner with reiki throughout the delivery.

Use with older people

Older people can also benefit from reiki. It should always be used, however, alongside conventional medicine, not as an alternative. Reiki practitioners need very little equipment so may be able to offer a mobile service for those that are housebound. Reiki can also be performed while the client is seated in a chair if necessary, meaning that it is accessible to all.

Case study

Here Sharon tells us about her experience with reiki:

'I had been ill for years and was fed up of feeling so lethargic. I'd suffered with glandular fever as a teenager and never fully recovered. I was diagnosed with ME or chronic fatigue syndrome as it is sometimes known. I went through periods of feeling totally exhausted and unable to function. During one of these periods I saw an advert from a reiki practitioner offering home visits. I was too weak to go out so thought that I should perhaps give it a try. I read up about reiki and was very sceptical about it, it didn't make any sense to me that it should work but I was desperate!

'At the first session the practitioner spoke to me about my condition and set up a couch in my living room. She drew the curtains and put on some relaxing music. I will admit I found it all a little bizarre and wanted to giggle, I was totally honest with her about how I felt and she acknowledged that most clients share this view at first. Once she started work I found that I had areas of my body that felt very warm. It was pleasurable and I felt deeply relaxed. The session lasted about 45 minutes and I didn't want it to end. When I sat up on the couch she passed me a mirror to look at myself. I couldn't believe it, the pale face that I'd had for months had disappeared and I could see the "old" me again. I continued to have sessions on a regular basis and decided that I should become attuned so that I could treat myself at home. Over time I went on to become attuned to masters level and while I don't practise on others I do use reiki for myself and my family. If others are thinking about trying reiki I would say, put aside your judgements and try it, you may get a surprise!'

What the experts say

Marion Eaton is a reiki master teacher from Hastings who has been practising reiki for over 16 years. She tells us, 'When looking for a reiki therapist the most important thing is the relationship between you and the practitioner. Make sure that you have a chat to them before committing to a session and go with your gut feelings about the practitioner. The best way to find a therapist is through personal recommendation.'

Reiki can be experienced differently by individuals. Marion says, 'Most people feel very relaxed and may even sleep when receiving reiki. Some clients comment on the warmth of my hands. If there is inflammation within the body, you may feel cold in these areas. Some people feel draughts, others small electric shock sensations and sometimes individuals see vivid colours. The experience varies with each session and for each individual. People tend to go away from the sessions feeling peaceful and calm and this feeling of tranquillity and wellbeing often continues for some time following the appointment.

'Reiki works where it is needed at the time and also works as is appropriate for the individual. It is important that you drink plenty of water following a session to help the reiki energy to push toxins out of the body. I always recommend that you are well-hydrated when you attend a reiki session and avoid drinking caffeine and alcohol prior to the appointment.'

For more information about Marion's work log on to her website at www.marioneaton.com and if you are interested in the reiki community see www.reikilights.net.

How to find a practitioner

The UK Reiki Federation have an online list of practitioners at www.reikifed. co.uk. Those included in the list have signed up to the organisation's code of ethics, have relevant insurance and hold appropriate certificates.

Quick action checklist

- Find your local practitioner.

- Read more about reiki.

- Speak to a reiki practitioner and find out about their work, whether they are insured and how their fees are structured.

Summing Up

Reiki is a natural healing therapy that works on many different levels. As it has progressed over time different styles of reiki have emerged. You may wish to ask your practitioner which style of reiki they use and to explain a little more about it to you.

Whatever the style, the method of receiving reiki is very simple and non-intrusive. Reiki can also be received at distance if you are unable to visit a practitioner. Reiki can be used alongside other treatments, for example a reflexologist may also be trained in reiki and use it during treatments.

Reiki is not an alternative to conventional medicine, but is very effective used alongside it.

Chapter Ten

Reflexology

Reflexology is the practice of applying pressure to certain parts of the feet, hands or ears in order to provide beneficial effects to other parts of the body. It is a natural healing system based on the premise that there are reflexes in the hands, ears and feet that relate to other areas of the body. By applying pressure to these reflexes, the functioning of those areas can be improved.

Foot reflexology is the most commonly practised form of reflexology. Some people imagine that it may tickle but firm pressure is used. The left foot corresponds to the left side of the body and the right foot to the right side. A reflexologist will treat both feet, even if you are only experiencing difficulties on one side of your body to ensure that you remain balanced.

When a particular part of the body is out of balance there may be a feeling of tenderness in the corresponding area of the foot. It is important that you share with the reflexologist if you feel any tender or sore spots during the treatment. Reflexology should not be used as a substitute for conventional medicine but can be used effectively alongside it. Energy blockages can be felt by the skilled practitioner, gentle but firm pressure will be applied to ease the congested area and to allow the energy to flow more freely.

If you don't fancy having your feet treated you can opt for hand or ear reflexology. Hand reflexology works in the same way as foot reflexology, although the reflex points are located more deeply. It can also be used when a foot is injured in some way. A reflexologist may show you where certain reflexes are in your hand so that you can use the techniques in-between appointments.

History

Reflexology dates back to ancient times. It is thought that reflexology was practised in China in 4000 BC and also in Ancient Egypt. A pictograph in the tomb of an Egyptian physician Ankhmahor (2500-2300 BC) shows two men working on the feet and hands of two others. The hieroglyphics state: 'Do not let it be painful'. The North American Indians have practised foot therapy for hundreds of years.

Dr William Fitzgerald called a systemised foot treatment 'zone therapy', which is an early form of reflexology. He found that if he exerted pressure on certain tips of the toes or fingers a corresponding part of the body would be anaesthetised. In 1915, Edwin Bowers wrote an article called: 'To stop that toothache, squeeze your toe'. This brought Dr Fitzgerald's work on zone therapy into the public forum. It remained a controversial subject in the medical world.

Eunice Ingham is known as the pioneer of reflexology, she devised a system of techniques for contacting the reflexes known as the 'Original Ingham Method'. Ingham produced a map of the entire body relating to specific areas on the feet. She devoted 40 years of her life to reflexology and helped to shape it into the practice that is performed today.

A typical treatment

As with the other therapies featured in this book, the first appointment will take longer than subsequent appointments. This is because a full consultation will take place which involves taking down your full medical history as well as discussing all areas of your lifestyle and wellbeing. You can expect the first session to last up to an hour and a half. You should also use this opportunity to ask any questions that you may have about the treatment. Follow-up treatments may last around 45 minutes to an hour. You can usually expect to see some results after four to six treatments, but ask your reflexologist if they are able to give you an indication as to how many sessions you are likely to need.

When receiving reflexology you will need to remove your socks or tights and your shoes. It is advisable to wear clothes that you feel comfortable in. Some reflexologists use a special chair that reclines, while others have a couch for you to lie on. An examination of both feet will take place and then the treatment will begin with some gentle massage to relax your foot. Some practitioners use creams, oils or talcum powder to work with, while others prefer to work directly onto your skin.

The reflexologist will then begin to work around your foot, covering each area with gentle pressure. Many people find this a relaxing experience and you may wish to close your eyes.

Following the treatment it is important to drink water in order to flush any toxins out of your system. You may experience a range of physical and emotional symptoms following the treatment, but these are short-lived and likely to be the result of the healing taking place within your body.

What is it used for?

Reflexology can be used for a variety of purposes including:

- Fertility issues.
- To promote relaxation and relieve stress.
- Improve circulation.
- Elimination of toxins.
- Promotion of the body's natural healing process.
- Calming the nervous system.

Contraindications

There are certain circumstances when reflexology should not be used. These include:

- Current risk of thrombosis (blood clots) or phlebitis.
- An unstable pregnancy.

- Certain types of cancer.
- Unstable heart conditions.

Some reflexologists may refer you back to your doctor if you are taking any prescription medication. If you have any concerns about whether reflexology is suitable for you, please speak to your reflexologist or discuss this with your GP before treatment begins.

Use with children

Children and babies can also benefit from the use of reflexology. Touch is very important to youngsters and can have a hugely positive effect on their wellbeing. A reflexologist may only treat a child for a short period of time due to their concentration span. Sometimes a few minutes is enough to see some benefit. Children generally respond quickly and positively to treatments. You may be shown how to use simple reflexology techniques at home with your child when visiting a practitioner.

Use with pregnant women

Reflexology can be used from conception and throughout pregnancy. In fact many women turn to reflexology if they are having difficulties conceiving – it may help you to relax, which in turn can help conception.

If you are considering using reflexology during pregnancy you should first consult your midwife. It should not be used if there is a history of premature labour, hypertension or recent vaginal bleeding. Some reflexologists do not treat women who are in their first trimester or at the end of their pregnancy, check when you contact them what their policy is on this.

Reflexology can help with many of the pregnancy niggles that women experience including:

- Backache.
- Nausea and sickness.
- Constipation.

- Fluid retention.

- Low energy levels.

- Anxiety.

There can also be benefits from receiving reflexology after the birth as it can help to rebalance the body.

Use with older people

Older people can enjoy reflexology, the caring contact that is given through reflexology can improve their emotional wellbeing. As a client only has to remove shoes and socks, it is a non-intrusive therapy that can be enjoyed in a sitting or lying position. There have been a number of studies carried out on the use of reflexology with older people and, while the results have varied, it has been found that it can be of both emotional and physical benefit. A reflexologist may be able to visit you at home to carry out the treatment.

Case study

David tells us about his experience of using reflexology:

'I visit a reflexologist on a weekly basis, I view it as my treat. I initially went to help with the irritable bowel syndrome that I suffer from and found that it did have positive results. I also found that it helped me to relax and reduced my feelings of anxiety. For this reason I continue to go on a regular basis and the treatment it is worth every penny. The only thing I would say to others considering reflexology is, if you can avoid driving afterwards, do. I like to get a lift home as I like to feel the continued benefit of the treatment; I find having to drive spoils it a little.'

What the experts say

Sarah Holland is an experienced reflexologist and runs her own practice in Hitchin, Hertfordshire. Here, she gives us some more information about reflexology, 'Check that your reflexologist has a relevant qualification and insurance for public liability. If you have a particular health condition it is worth asking what experience they have working with it.

'Reflexology is suitable for virtually anyone, from tiny babies to older people. It can be used alongside conventional medicine or as a stand-alone therapy. Many people first try reflexology when they have a health problem that they can't resolve, while others have reflexology purely for relaxation.

'Reflexology is not yet available on the NHS, although is offered in some health authorities, often in cancer care or maternity wards. The majority of people will have reflexology from a private therapist and fund the treatment themselves, although there are some health policies that will reimburse treatments.

'Reflexology is often used for conditions that the medical world can find no cause for and no treatment that really works. Typically these can be stress-related conditions, such as irritable bowel syndrome, migraine, chronic fatigue syndrome/ME. Clients often gain positive results when using reflexology to treat these conditions.

'Finally it's not ticklish and the reflexologist really won't mind your misshapen feet or hairy toes! These are people's main worries when they come to see me!'

Marian is one of Sarah's clients and tells us, 'After many years of severe and regular migraine attacks I decided to try reflexology, and was totally amazed by the results. I look forward to my treatments so much, they are a real treat, and so relaxing. My migraines are now under control and I feel that reflexology has transformed my life.'

Visit Sarah's website at www.sarah-holland.co.uk.

How to find a practitioner

The Association of Reflexologists (AoR) is an independent body that provides support for qualified and training practitioners. By visiting the website you can find a reflexologist in your area www.aor.org.uk. Those that are registered will use 'MAR' after their names which stands for Member of the Association of Reflexologists. This indicates that these individuals are trained to the standards agreed with the AoR. When finding a practitioner you should ask about their insurance and also establish what the cost of your treatment is likely to be.

Quick action checklist

- Find out more about how each area of your foot or hand corresponds to parts of your body. There are many books about reflexology that you can read, or maps of the feet and hands are readily available on the Internet.

- Find out if there is a qualified practitioner in your area by visiting the Association of Reflexologists' website.

- Ask others about their experience of reflexology.

Summing Up

Reflexology is the act of placing pressure on specific points in the hands, feet or ears, in order to facilitate a physical change in the body. Reflexology charts provide us with a map of the feet and hands and indicate which specific part relates to what part of the body. For example, the ball of the foot mirrors the chest and upper back as well as the heart and the lungs.

Reflexology can reduce stress levels and help the body to become more balanced which in turn can benefit the immune system. Further scientific study needs to be carried out in order to come to some conclusive results as to whether reflexology can help with specific illness and disease.

A reflexologist cannot diagnose conditions and reflexology should be used alongside conventional medicine rather than as a replacement for it.

Help List

General information

Complementary and Natural Healthcare Council (CNHC)

83 Victoria Street, London, SW1H 0HW
www.cnhc.org.uk
The UK regulator for complementary healthcare practitioners. Check the online
register to find registered practitioners.

Acupuncture

Acupuncture Resource Research Centre (ARRC)

Faculty of Health and Human Sciences, Thames Valley University, Paragon
House, Boston, Manor Road, Brentford, Middlesex, TW8 9GA
Tel: 020 8209 4277
www.acupunctureresearch.org.uk
ARRC is a specialist resource for acupuncture research information funded
by the British Acupuncture Council and hosted by Thames Valley University's
Centre for Complementary Healthcare and Integrated Medicine (CCHIM).

British Acupuncture Council (BAcC)

63 Jeddo Road, London, W12 9HQ
Tel: 020 8735 0400
Fax: 020 8735 0404
www.acupuncture.org.uk
The UK's largest professional body for acupuncturists. Log on to the website
to find a registered practitioner.

May Stevens

Pampered Clinic, 673 Abbeydale Rd, Sheffield, S7 2BE
Tel: 0114 250 7617
Sheffield Therapy Centre, 500 Ridgeway Rd, Gleadless, S12 2JX
Tel: 0114 239 0022
Tel: 07773 316 108
maystevensacupuncture@gmail.com
www.maystevensacupuncture.co.uk
Acupuncturist based in Sheffield.

Aromatherapy

Aromatherapy Council

www.aromatherapycouncil.org
The lead body for the aromatherapy profession in the UK. Provides a list of qualified aromatherapists.

Chiropractic

British Chiropractic Council

59 Castle Street, Reading, Berkshire, RG1 7SN
Tel: 0118 950 5950
enquiries@chiropractic-uk.co.uk
www.chiropractic-uk.co.uk
The British Chiropractic Council is the largest and longest established association for chiropractors in the UK. Their website allows you to do a postcode search to find your nearest chiropractor.

General Chiropractic Council (GCC)

44 Wicklow Street, London, WC1X 9HL
Tel: 020 7713 5155
www.gcc-uk.org

All chiropractors in the UK must be registered with the GCC. The Council check chiropractors who apply for registration to make sure that they have a suitable qualification and are of sound character.

Herbal medicine

Association of Master Herbalists

www.associationofmasterherbalists.co.uk
Search for local practitioners using this website.

Ayurvedic Practitioners Association (APA)

www.apa.uk.com
APA is committed to supporting all Ayurvedic professionals in the UK. You can search for a practitioner on their website.

European Herbal and Traditional Medicine Practitioners Association

http://ehtpa.eu
The EHTPA is an umbrella body which represents professional associations of herbal/traditional medicine practitioners offering variously western herbal medicine, Chinese herbal medicine, Ayurveda and traditional Tibetan medicine.

Foreman and Jones

Integrated Health Practice, 112d High Street, Hythe, Kent, CT21 5LE
www.foremanandjonesherbaldispensary.co.uk
http://twitter.com/ForemanandJones
Facebook: ForemanandJones HerbsandHypnotherapy
Tel: 01303 760001
Visit the website for natural products, or if you live in Kent you can visit for a consultation.

Medicines and Healthcare Products Regulatory Agency

Market Towers, 1 Nine Elms Lane, London, SW8 5NQ
Tel: 020 7084 2000
www.mhra.gov.uk
Regulates new and existing pharmaceutical products, including herbal medicines, and medical equipment.

National Institute of Medical Herbalists

Elm House, 54 Mary Arches Street, Exeter, EX4 3BA
Tel: 01392 426022
www.nimh.org.uk
Use this website to find details of your local medical herbalists.

Register of Chinese Herbal Medicine (RCHM)

Office 5, 1 Exeter Street, Norwich, NR2 4QB
Tel: 01603 623994
Fax: 01603 667557
herbmed@rchm.co.uk
www.rchm.co.uk
RCHM works with Chinese herbal medicine practitioners to ensure codes of practice are followed.

The College of Practitioners of Phytotherapy

Oak Glade, 9 Hythe Close, Polegate, East Sussex, BN26 6LQ
Telephone: 01323 484353
pamela.bull@phytotherapists.org
www.phytotherapists.org
Aims to bring together professional herbalists, you can search for practitioners on the website.

Unified Register of Herbal Practitioners

www.urhp.com
Provides a comprehensive register of qualified and insured herbal practitioners who offer the public high quality herbal medicine treatment from many traditions.

Homeopathy

Karen Runacres

DL Ogle Ltd, 18-20 St Johns, Worcester, Worcestershire, WR2 5AH
Tel: 01905 428 028
www.homeopathyworcester.co.uk
Homeopath based in Worcestershire, Karen is registered with The Society of
Homeopaths.

The Society of Homeopaths

11 Brookfield, Duncan Close, Moulton Park, Northampton, NN3 6WL
Tel: 0845 450 6611
www.homeopathy-soh.org
The Society of Homeopaths has a list of practitioners who have met with
their professional standard and practice in accordance with their ethics. The
homeopaths listed also have full professional and indemnity insurance.

Hypnotherapy

Cambridge College of Hypnotherapy (CCH)

CCH Ltd Office, 24 Milton Road, Impington, Cambridge, CB24 9NF
Tel: 01223 235 127
j.teague@ntlworld.com
www.hypnotherapytraining.org.uk
Training college for hypnotherapy.

General Hypnotherapy Register (GHR)

PO Box 204, Lymington, SO41 6DH
Tel: 01590 683770
admin@general-hypnotherapy-register.com
www.general-hypnotherapy-register.com
The GHR is the largest professional register of hypnotherapists in the UK.

Hypnotherapy Society

PO Box 131, Arundel, BN18 8BR
Tel: 0870 8503387
secretary@hypnotherapysociety.com
www.hypnotherapysociety.com
To find a hypnotherapist you may wish to check those that are a member of the Hypnotherapy Society by logging on to their website.

Hypnotherapy Training Institute

www.hypnotherapy.com
Information on becoming a trained hypnotherapist.

Lynn Wilshaw/Hippo Hypno

The Sycamores, 1 Racecourse Close, Swinton, Mexborough, South Yorkshire, S64 8EW
Tel: 01709 875 475
www.lynnwilshaw.co.uk
www.hippohypno.co.uk
Hypnotherapist based in South Yorkshire. Hippo Hypno is an online store selling hypnotherapy CDs for use at home.

Massage

General Council for Massage Therapies (GCMT)

27 Old Gloucester Street, London, WC1N 3XX
Tel: 0870 850 4452
www.gcmt.org.uk
The governing body for massage therapists in the UK. It can also help you to find a practitioner by visiting the website.

International Association of Infant Massage (IAIM)

Unit 10, Marlborough Business Centre, 96 George Lane, South Woodford,
London, E18 1AD
Tel: 020 8989 9597
www.iaim.org.uk
The IAIM can also provide you with details of local practitioners and classes if
you visit the website.

Marion Eaton

Whisperwood, New Cut, Westfield, Hastings, TN35 4RD
Tel: 01424 755401
07804358815
www.marioneaton.com
www.marioneaton.org.uk
Marion is an experienced therapist from Hastings who is trained in Swedish
massage, holistic massage, professional aromatherapy, and NO HANDS
massage®.

Massage Therapy UK

www.massagetherapy.co.uk
Massage Therapy UK provides information about massage and has a directory
of practitioners that can be searched online.

Rakhee Shah

www.haveamassage.co.uk
Rakhee is based in New Barnet, Hertfordshire and carries out a number of
different types of massage, including Indian head massage.

Osteopathy

British Osteopathic Association

3 Park Terrace, Manor Road, Luton, Beds, LU1 3HN
Tel: 01582 488455
www.osteopathy.org
Search the online directory to find an osteopath.

British School of Osteopathy

275 Borough High Street, London, SE1 1JE
www.bso.ac.uk
Offers training for osteopaths. You may be able to get access to affordable osteopathic care through one of its clinics.

General Osteopathic Council (GOsC)

176 Tower Bridge Road, London, SE1 3LU
Tel: 020 7357 6655
contactus@osteopathy.org.uk
www.osteopathy.org.uk
The GOsC regulates the practice of osteopathy in the UK.

Jane Jeater

www.janejeater.co.uk
Jane provides osteopath services to Hastings, Battle, Hawkhurst, and the surrounding East Sussex and Kent area.

Lin Bridgeford

Saltdean Practice, 108 Rodmell Ave, Saltdean, Brighton, BN2 8PJ
Tel: 07710 227 038
01273 309 557
osteopathy@osteo-info.co.uk
www.osteo-info.co.uk
An experienced osteopath based in Brighton.

Osteopathic Sports Care Association (OSCA)

1 Brewers Yard, Ivel Road, Shefford, Bedfordshire, SG17 5GY
Tel: 07807 356 485
secretary@osca.org.uk
www.osca.org.uk
The OSCA website can help you find an osteopath with a special interest in treating sports injuries.

Mark Pitcairn-Knowles

Springbank Clinic, 13 Pembroke Road, Sevenoaks, TN13 1XR
Tel: 01732 453956
www.SpringbankClinic.co.uk
Mark is an experienced osteopath and principal of the Springbank Clinic.

Sutherland Cranial College

Stuart House, The Back, Chepstow, NP16 5HH
Tel: 01291 622555
www.sutherlandcranialcollege.co.uk
To find a cranial osteopath log on to the website.

Reiki

Marion Eaton

www.marioneaton.com
Reiki practitioner and reiki master.

Reiki Lights

www.reikilights.net
An online community where you can find out more about reiki.

The UK Reiki Federation

PO Box 71, Andover, SP11 9WQ
Tel: 01264 791441
www.reikifed.co.uk
The federation can provide a list of reiki practitioners who have signed up to their code of ethics.

Reflexology

Sarah Holland

71 Whitehill Road, Hitchin, Herts, SG4 9HP
Tel: 01462 621393
www.sarah-holland.co.uk
Sarah is a reflexologist based in Hertfordshire.

The Association of Reflexologists

5 Fore Street, Taunton, Somerset, TA1 1HX
www.aor.org.uk
The Association of Reflexologists is an independent body that provides
support for qualified and training practitioners

References

UK Back Pain Exercise and Manipulation trial, MRC, 'United Kingdom Back Pain Exercise and Manipulation (UK BEAM) randomised trial: effectiveness of physical treatments for back pain in primary care', BMJ, 2004, doi:10.1136/bmj.38282.669225.AE.

Licciardone *et al.*, 'Osteopathic manipulative treatment for low back pain: a systematic review and meta-analysis of randomized controlled trials'. BMC Musculoskelet Disord, vol. 6, 2005, doi: 10.1186/1471-2474-6-43. PMID 16080794.

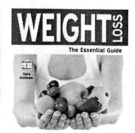
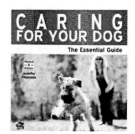
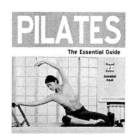
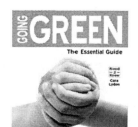
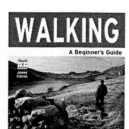

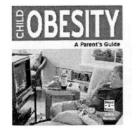
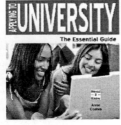
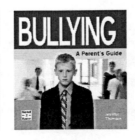
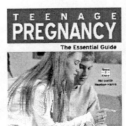
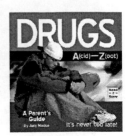